Copyright - 2022 -

All rights reserved.

This document is geared towards providing exact and reliable information in regard to the topic and issue covered.

- From a Declaration of Principles which was accepted and approved equally by a Committee of the American Bar Association and a Committee of Publishers and Associations.

In no way is it legal to reproduce, duplicate, or transmit any part of this document in either electronic means or in printed format. All rights reserved.

The information provided herein is stated to be truthful and consistent, in that any liability, in terms of inattention or otherwise, by any usage or abuse of any policies, processes, or directions contained within is the solitary and utter responsibility of the recipient reader. Under no circumstances will any legal responsibility or blame be held against the publisher for any reparation, damages, or monetary loss due to the information herein, either directly or indirectly.

Respective authors own all copyrights not held by the publisher.

The information herein is offered for informational purposes solely and is universal as so. The presentation of the information is without contract or any type of guarantee assurance.

The trademarks that are used are without any consent, and the publication of the trademark is without permission or backing by the trademark owner. All trademarks and brands within this book are for clarifying purposes only and are owned by the owners themselves, not affiliated with this document.

TABLE OF CONTENTS

DASH DIET   12

INTRODUCTION   14

CHAPTER 1   18
WHAT IS THE DASH DIET?
What is the Dash Diet?
Concepts of the Dash Diet
Beginning of the DASH Diet

CHAPTER 2   30
BENEFITS OF THE DASH DIET
Controlled Blood Pressure 30
Healthy Eating
Reduced Risk of Osteoporosis
Healthy Cholesterol Levels
Better Weight Management
Healthier Kidneys
Easy to Maintain
Prevents Diabetes
Decreased Risk of Certain Cancers
Better Mental Health
You Feel Less Hungry
Healthy Lifestyle
Anti-Aging Properties
Improved Cognitive Function
Reduced Risk of Developing Heart Disease

CHAPTER 3   36
28 DAY MEAL PLAN
Week 1

Week 2
Week 3
Week 4

CHAPTER 4 — 42
SHOPPING LIST
Week 1
Week 2
Week 3
Week 4

CHAPTER 5 — 48
MEAL PLAN WEEK 1

Day 1 — 48
Breakfast - Avocado Cup with Egg
Lunch - Garlic Mushroom Chicken
Dinner - Easy Beef Brisket

Day 2 — 52
Breakfast - Greek Yogurt Oat Pancakes
Lunch - Chicken Wrap
Dinner - Baked Fish Served with Vegetables

Day 3 — 55
Breakfast - Brown Sugar Cinnamon Oatmeal
Lunch - Tuna Sandwich
Dinner - Paella with Chicken, Leeks, and Tarragon

Day 4 — 60
Breakfast - Almond Butter-Banana Smoothie
Lunch - Tofu & Green Bean Stir-Fry
Dinner - Salsa Chicken Chili

Day 5 — 63
Breakfast - Savory Yogurt Bowls
Lunch - Italian Stuffed Portobello Mushroom Burgers
Dinner - Chicken with Mushrooms

Day 6 66
    Breakfast - Oatmeal Banana Pancakes with Walnuts
    Lunch - Curry Vegetable Noodles with Chicken
    Dinner - Olive Capers Chicken

Day 7 70
    Breakfast - Sweet Berries Pancake
    Lunch - Black Bean Stew with Cornbread
    Dinner - Southwestern Chicken and Pasta

CHAPTER 6 73
MEAL PLAN WEEK 2

Day 8 73
    Breakfast - Carrot Muffins
    Lunch - Eggplant Parmesan Stacks
    Dinner - Beef Stew with Fennel and Shallots

Day 9 78
    Breakfast - Pumpkin Muffins
    Lunch - Dill and Lemon Cod Packets
    Dinner - Stuffed Chicken Breasts

Day 10 81
    Breakfast - Apple Pancakes
    Lunch - Salmon Wrap
    Dinner - Honey Crusted Chicken

Day 11 84
    Breakfast - Strawberry Sandwich
    Lunch - Sweet Potatoes and Zucchini Soup
    Dinner - Pork and Roasted Tomatoes Mix

Day 12 87
    Breakfast - Scrambled Egg and Veggie Breakfast Quesadillas
    Lunch - Chickpea Cauliflower Tikka Masala
    Dinner - Easy Shrimp

Day 13 90
    Breakfast - Energy Sunrise Muffins
    Lunch - Mexican-Style Potato Casserole

Dinner - Basil Halibut

Day 14   94

Breakfast - Creamy Oats & Blueberry Smoothie

Lunch - Dill Chicken Salad

Dinner - White Beans with Spinach and Pan-Roasted Tomatoes

CHAPTER 7   97

MEAL PLAN WEEK 3

Day 15   97

Breakfast - Spinach, Egg, and Cheese Breakfast Quesadillas

Lunch - Sweet and Sour Chicken Whit Noodles and Vegetable

Dinner - Leek & Cauliflower Soup

Day 16   104

Breakfast - Blueberry Waffles

Lunch - Steamed Salmon Teriyaki

Dinner - Pork Medallions with Five Spice Powder

Day 17   107

Breakfast - Super-Simple Granola

Lunch - Light Balsamic Salad

Dinner - Mustard Chicken Tenders

Day 18   110

Breakfast - Breakfast Banana Split

Lunch - Lemongrass and Chicken Soup

Dinner - Spicy Cod

Day 19   113

Breakfast - Breakfast Fruits Bowls

Lunch - Fruited Quinoa Salad

Dinner - Grilled Pork Fajitas

Day 20   116

Breakfast - Easy Veggie Muffins

Lunch - Easy Lunch Salmon Steaks

Dinner - Provence Pork Medallions

Day 21   120

Breakfast - Mushrooms and Cheese Omelet

Lunch - White Chicken Chili
Dinner - Coconut Shrimp

CHAPTER 8   123
MEAL PLAN WEEK 4

Day 22   123
Breakfast - Apple Quinoa Muffins
Lunch - Easy Steamed Alaskan Cod
Dinner - Simple Beef Brisket and Tomato Soup

Day 23   128
Breakfast - Steel Cut Oat Blueberry Pancakes
Lunch - Pork and Dates Sauce
Dinner - Fish in a Vegetable Patch

Day 24   131
Breakfast - Pineapple Oatmeal
Lunch - Sweet Potato-Turkey Meatloaf
Dinner - Steamed Blue Crabs

Day 25   134
Breakfast - Banana & Cinnamon Oatmeal
Lunch - Turkey Wrap
Dinner - Asian Salmon

Day 26   138
Breakfast - Zucchini Pancakes
Lunch - White Beans Stew
Dinner - Garlic Pepper Chicken

Day 27   141
Breakfast - Carrot Cake Overnight Oats
Lunch - Spicy Tofu Burrito Bowls with Cilantro Avocado Sauce
Dinner - Baked Chicken

Day 28   144
Breakfast - Egg White Breakfast Mix
Lunch - Chicken with Potatoes Olives & Sprouts
Dinner - Ginger Sesame Salmon

CONCLUSION — **147**

KEEP COOKING TASTY AND HEALTHY RECIPES AFTER YOU FINISH YOUR MEAL PLAN, MORE THAN 99 RECIPES AT YOUR DISPOSAL SO YOU CAN INDULGE YOURSELF AND HAVE FUN WITH YOUR WHOLE FAMILY!

CHAPTER 9 — **150**
SMOOTHIE RECIPES

1. Creamy Apple-Avocado Smoothie — 150
2. Strawberry, Orange, and Beet Smoothie — 151
3. Mixed Berries Smoothie — 152
4. Satisfying Berry and Almond Smoothie — 153
5. Refreshing Mango and Pear Smoothie — 154
6. Blackberry and Apple Smoothie — 155
7. Mint Flavored Pear Smoothie — 156
8. Chilled Watermelon Smoothie — 157
9. Blueberry-Vanilla Yogurt Smoothie — 158
10. Banana-Peanut Butter and Greens Smoothie — 159

CHAPTER 10 — **162**
BREAKFAST RECIPES

11. Very Berry Muesli — 162
12. Sweet Potato Toast Three Ways — 163
13. Steel-Cut Oatmeal with Plums and Pear — 164
14. French Toast with Applesauce — 165
15. Breakfast Hash — 166
16. Chia Seeds Breakfast Mix — 167
17. Breakfast Fruits Bowls — 168
18. Pumpkin Cookies — 169
19. Veggie Scramble — 171
20. Pesto Omelet — 171
21. Bagels Made Healthy — 172

22. Cereal with Cranberry-Orange Twist — 173
23. No Cook Overnight Oats — 174
24. Simple Cheese and Broccoli Omelets — 175
25. Creamy Avocado and Egg Salad Sandwiches — 176

CHAPTER 11 — 178
LUNCH RECIPES

26. Stuffed Eggplant Shells — 178
27. Southwestern Vegetables Tacos — 179
28. Seared Scallops with Blood Orange Glaze — 180
29. Lemon Garlic Shrimp — 181
30. Shrimp Fra Diavolo — 182
31. Fish Amandine — 183
32. Lemon Salmon with Kaffir Lime — 184
33. Pork Roast and Cranberry Roast — 185
34. Easy Pork Chops — 186
35. Ground Beef with Greens & Tomatoes — 187
36. Curried Beef Meatballs — 188
37. Chicken Thighs and Apples Mix — 189
38. Thai Chicken Thighs — 190
39. Falling "Off" The Bone Chicken — 191
40. Garlic Pork Shoulder — 192
41. Grilled Flank Steak with Lime Vinaigrette — 193
42. Asian Pork Tenderloin — 194
43. Simple Beef Brisket and Tomato Soup — 195
44. Rustic Beef and Barley Soup — 196
45. Southwestern Bean Salad with Creamy Avocado Dressing — 197
46. Cobb Pasta Salad — 198
47. Edamame Salad with Corn and Cranberries — 199
48. Warm Asian Slaw — 200
49. Tangy Three-Bean Salad with Barley — 201
50. Tuna Salad-Stuffed Tomatoes with Arugula — 202
51. Steamed Veggie and Lemon Pepper Salmon — 203
52. Steamed Fish with Scallions and Ginger — 204

53. Steamed Tilapia with Green Chutney	205
54. Creamy Haddock with Kale	206
55. Stewed Cod Filet with Tomatoes	207

CHAPTER 12 — 210
SNACK RECIPES

56. Mini Teriyaki Turkey Sandwiches	210
57. Peach Crumble Muffins	211
58. Peanut Butter Banana Bread Bites	212
59. Toasted Almond Ambrosia	213
60. Zesty Zucchini Muffins	214
61. Blueberry Oat Muffins	215
62. Banana Bread	216
63. Milk Chocolate Pudding	217
64. Minty Lime and Grapefruit Yogurt Parfait	218
65. Peach Tarts	219
66. Raspberry Nuts Parfait	220
67. Apricot Biscotti	221
68. Apple & Berry Cobbler	222
69. Mixed Fruit Compote Cups	223
70. Generous Garlic Bread Stick	224

CHAPTER 13 — 226
DINNER RECIPES

71. Sweet-Ginger Scallops	226
72. Savory Lobster Roll	227
73. Garlic and Tomatoes on Mussels	228
74. Oven-Fried Chicken Breasts	229
75. Rosemary Roasted Chicken	230
76. Artichoke and Spinach Chicken	231
77. Pumpkin and Black Beans Chicken	232
78. Spicy Lamb Curry	233
79. Ground Lamb with Harissa	234
80. Pan-Seared Lamb Chops	235
81. Lamb & Pineapple Kebabs	236

82. Spiced Pork One	237
83. Vegetable Cheese Calzone	238
84. Mixed Vegetarian Chili	239
85. Coconut Curry Sea Bass	240
86. Zucchini Pepper Kebabs	241
87. Asparagus Cheese Vermicelli	242
88. Pesto Chicken Breasts with Summer Squash	243
89. Chicken, Tomato and Green Beans	244
90. Chicken Tortillas	245
91. Roast and Mushrooms	246
92. Pork and Celery Mix	247
93. Corn Stuffed Peppers	248
94. Black Bean Soup	249
95. Chickpea & Kale Soup	250
96. Clam Chowder	251
97. Honey Spiced Cajun Chicken	252
98. Italian Chicken	253
99. Lemon-Parsley Chicken Breast	254
100. Currant Pork Chops	255
CONCLUSION	**257**
INDEX	**259**

DASH DIET

THE COMPLETE GUIDE FOR BEGINNERS WITH A COMPLETE 28 DAYS MEAL PLAN. INEXPENSIVE, QUICK, EASY, AND HEALTHY LOW-SODIUM RECIPES TO LOWER YOUR BLOOD PRESSURE

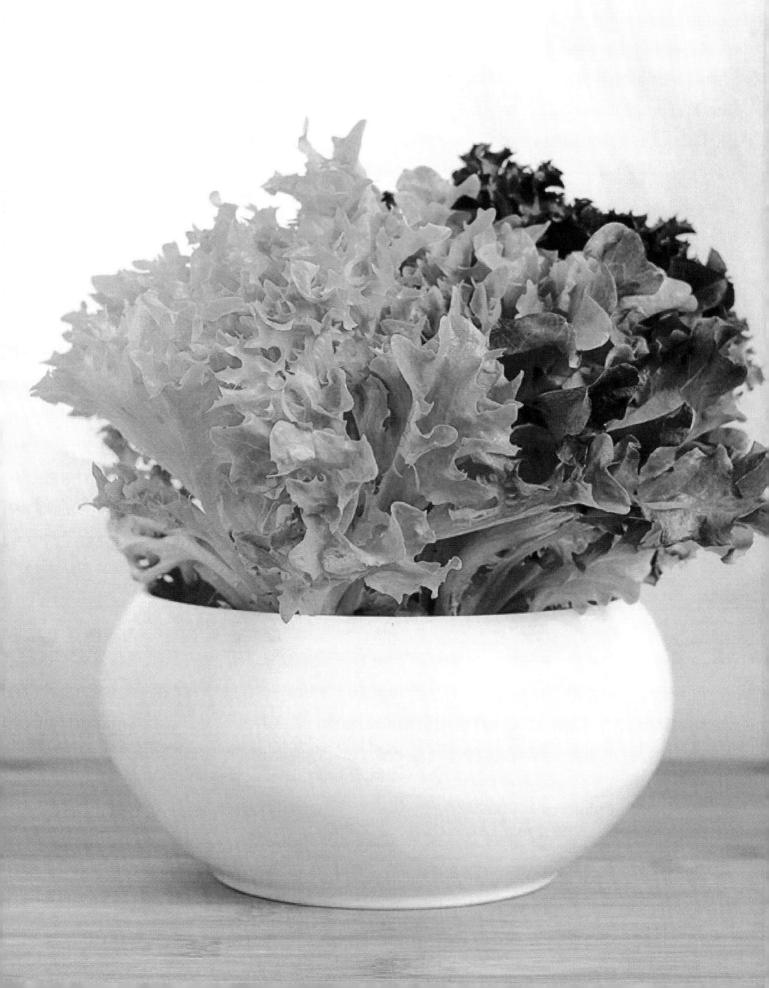

INTRODUCTION

The DASH diet is a powerful means to help people with heart disease and high blood pressure regain balance, improve their lives, and take control of their health. DASH diet is also a weight reduction diet that depends upon the proportions in which the food is consumed.

The most important thing about this diet is that it doesn't restrict any food groups.

Some consider this diet plan costly, but if you look at it from another angle, you'll see that it can save thousands of dollars that would otherwise be spent on expensive medications.

Consequently, the dash diet brings better health and is also an economical and long-term solution to avoid many kinds of health problems.

The dash diet has a lot of health benefits both directly and indirectly. The thrust of this diet is to have total health that directly affects physical and mental wellbeing. This diet doesn't put any restrictions on consumption. Instead, the dash diet encourages its consumers to have more and more with a little concentration.

Moreover, a low-carb diet also acts like a magic wand to balance blood pressure, sugar, and cholesterol levels. The consumption of strong and healthy food gives strength, energy, and vitality to the human body. In this cookbook, you will find all the recipes you need to enjoy a delicious, flavorful, and simple DASH diet. Whether you are looking for a quick and easy meal or something special to celebrate an important holiday or milestone, these recipes will be your go-to. These recipes can be shared with friends and loved ones over a table with laughter and joy, allowing you to truly enjoy the experience of a delicious meal. Whether you are together with loved ones or alone, these meals will offer you comfort. Along with the recipes in this book is a shopping list, 28-day meal plan with the nutritional index of each recipe.

Please remember, I am not a doctor, and this book is not making medical claims or practicing medicine. You should always discuss anything related to medicine, health, or diet with your doctor before making any changes. This applies to all of the information in this book.

DASH DIET 2022

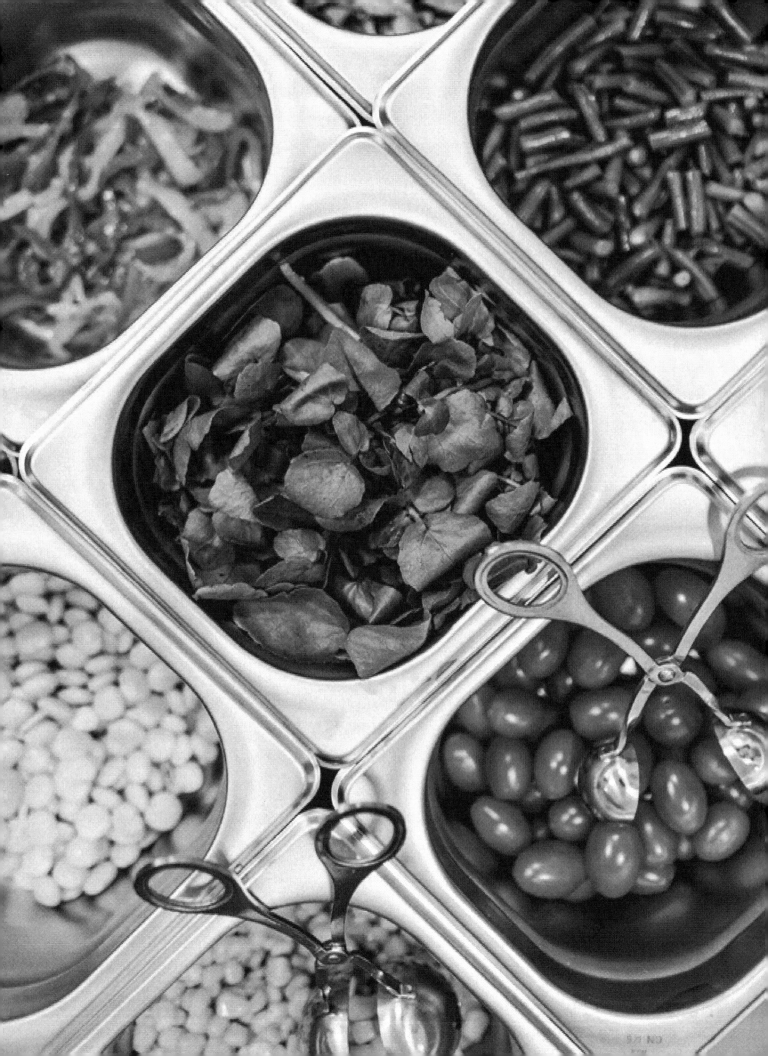

CHAPTER 1

WHAT IS THE DASH DIET?

Unlike the regular diets out there, DASH is a tad bit different. It means Dietary Approaches to Stop Hypertension. Yes, you read that right. Finally, a diet that focuses on one of the greatest killers of the 21st century—hypertension. According to recent studies, one out of three adults suffers from hypertension or high blood pressure. It keeps increasing with age, with almost two-thirds of the population suffering from it from the age of 65. High blood pressure is not a single stroke disease—it brings heart trouble, kidney diseases, and even diabetes.

Our sedentary lifestyles, coupled with unhealthy eating habits, have fueled several hypertension-related diseases. Most can be corrected by following a healthy diet, which is what DASH aims at. This diet comprises foods and recipes that promote lower sodium levels and higher potassium, calcium, fiber, and magnesium levels in the body. It also helps lower the overall blood pressure to an optimum level without harming the body's processes. When this happens, disorders related to hypertension disappear, such as osteoporosis, diabetes, and kidney failure.

The original diet plan aimed to lower blood pressure through natural foods and without medication aid. It was sponsored and endorsed by the US National Institute of Health. When the first DASH diet trials came out, it was found that lowering the blood pressure helped maintain the level even with some excess sodium in the blood. Not only this, but the diet was also beneficial in keeping the extra pounds off and preventing many disorders related to hypertension.

WHO SHOULD FOLLOW THIS DIET?

Is the diet for me? Or is it only for people with existing hypertension problems? According to the Dietary Guidelines for Americans, the DASH diet is a healthy eating model that anyone can follow. Of course, since the diet's primary objective is to lower blood pressure, people suffering from hypertension become the primary beneficiaries of the diet. But anyone who wishes to get healthy and scientifically lose weight can follow it, children included.

This diet works while other diets fail miserably because the body is kept full with the required nutrition. The fundamental nutrients, such as calcium, magnesium, and potassium, are elevated in the body through a wholesome diet plan, and sodium levels are also kept in control. And it is all done in a controlled, scientific, and disciplined manner without any crashes or spikes in the metabolism, ensuring a healthier you.

CONCEPTS OF THE DASH DIET

The Dash diet is based on the following principles:

1. Reduction in—salt consumption

One of the main goals of the Dash diet is to reduce the consumption of salt drastically. Of course, man cannot live without salt. The human body contains around 150 to 300 grams of table salt. Therefore, the amount of salt lost through sweating and other excretions must be replaced. Salt supports bone structure and digestion. It maintains the osmotic pressure in the vessels to maintain the water and nutrient levels. But nowadays our foods are filled with a lot of salt—especially all finished products.

The extent to which increased salt consumption has a negative impact on health is currently the subject of intense discussion among experts, especially since the body excretes excess salt.

But studies from 1970 in Finland already show that too much salt causes blood pressure to skyrocket. It could be demonstrated that the reduced consumption of salt by 30% could even reduce mortality from heart attacks by 80%.

A study on mice published in 2007 at the University Hospital in Heidelberg showed that a lot of salt increases blood pressure: *"Salt promotes the formation of certain messenger substances in the muscles of blood vessels that cause the muscle cells to contract. The increased resistance in the blood vessels increases blood pressure"*. Therefore, Heidelberg scientists see considerable advantages in reducing the amount of salt in food compared to conventional drugs.

There is disagreement among scientists about how high the maximum amount of salt can be. While US experts recommend a maximum of 1.5 grams of salt per day, the German Nutrition Society's recommendation is 6 grams per day. The upper limit is 10 grams per day. Six grams are roughly equivalent to a teaspoon.

However, this only applies to a healthy person who moves sufficiently and is physically active and excretes the salt again through sweating. For example, an athlete can tolerate more salt than someone who only moves moderately.

I recommend that you only look at these values as a rough guide and begin to control your salt consumption and gradually reduce it. Also, keep in mind that the maximum amount of salt you should consume depends on your body constitution and lifestyle.

Recommendation:

- Less is more! Therefore, pay more attention to your salt consumption in the future and reduce it step by step. The keyword is **low-salt, but not salt-free!**

- Avoid finished products (packaged food, pizza, French fries, chips, canned food, various meat and fish products, baked goods, etc.). If necessary, read the list of ingredients.

- If possible, use a **natural salt substitute** (herbs, etc.) in your meals.

- Use **low-water cooking methods**, such as stewing or steaming. This means that the food remains tastier, and you don't need to salt it as much.

2. More vitamin E and minerals

The Dash diet is based on a variety of fruits and vegetables and whole-grain products to provide the body with plenty of vitamins and minerals. Particular attention is paid to minerals such as magnesium and potassium, which help lower or improve blood pressure.

3. More healthy fats and oils

Fats are energy carriers and ensure that fat-soluble vitamins such as vitamins E, D, and K can be absorbed by the body at all. Certain fatty acids, such as omega-3 and omega-6 fatty acids, are also essential, meaning we can only get them from food. Therefore, they should be on a regular meal plan. The omega-6/3 ratio plays a vital role in health. **Omega-3 fatty** acids help to maintain normal blood pressure levels wisely. However, our diet often contains too little omega-3 fatty acids. Good sources of this are **fatty fish** such as herring, mackerel, salmon, and sardines.

This also applies to the use of oils. Z and healthy oils include virgin cold-pressed **olive oil and coconut oil** (in organic quality).

Unlike olive oil, coconut oil can also be heated and used for frying and baking. On the other hand, the much-used sunflower oil is less healthy because it only contains omega-6 fatty acids. This creates an imbalance in the omega-3 to omega-6 ratio. A ratio between 1:2 and 1: 5 should be aimed for.

Ultimately, as with most other diets, the Dash diet should avoid unhealthy fats, especially trans fats, a subgroup of unsaturated fatty acids, and replace them with healthy fats such as those found in nuts, seeds, and fish. Trans fatty acids come from industrial production and are, for example, contained in chips, baked goods, French fries, confectionery, pizza, etc.

4. More fiber

Fiber is an integral part of the Dash diet. A fiber-rich diet positively affects blood pressure and the cardiovascular system, whether through fruits, vegetables, grains, or cereals.

Therefore, in contrast to the low-carb diet, grain can be

consumed. However, it is essential to consume only **wholesome grains** (whole grain bread).

5. Egg whites/proteins

Proteins are an essential part of the Dash diet and should be consumed in beans, lentils, fish, and soy products.

6. White instead of dark meat

Animal fat should be avoided as far as possible. It is high in cholesterol and saturated fat. Therefore, red meat should be avoided entirely if possible. Instead, white meat (chicken, turkey) can be put on the plate.

7. Avoid butter

Even if opinions differ widely about butter consumption, especially its effect on cholesterol, the Dash diet specifies that butter should be avoided as far as possible. Therefore, butter no longer belongs in the refrigerator. Vegetable oils should serve as a substitute.

Now margarine is anything but healthy and therefore not an alternative in my opinion. Therefore, recommend switching to ghee, the Ayurvedic butter. Ghee is pure butterfat and contains 70% saturated fatty acids. In Ayurveda, Ghee has been used for healing purposes for thousands of years. Studies have shown that ghee can even lower cholesterol and prevent diseases such as cardiovascular diseases. The advantage of ghee is that, unlike butter, it can be heated to a high temperature.

8. Low-fat dairy products

The reduced-fat variant should always be preferred for dairy products (max. 1.5% fat content).

9. Less alcohol, caffeine, and nicotine

Alcohol increases blood pressure. The Dash diet recommends avoiding alcohol, beverages containing caffeine, and nicotine as much as possible to reduce blood pressure.

If you don't want to go without your coffee, you should enjoy it with as little or no sugar as possible. It is also known that smoking increases the risk of heart attacks and strokes. So, if you haven't already done so—put an end to the glowing stick!

10. Reduction of industrial sugar (granulated sugar)

Most people should know by now that too much sugar is not healthy. The Dash diet does not completely exclude sugar. After all, fresh and dried fruits are an important part of this diet, and of course, they also contain sugar (fructose).

However, what has a negative effect on blood pressure is pure industrial sugar. This can quickly increase blood pressure and should be avoided as far as possible. The best way to regulate daily sugar consumption is to avoid sweets and finished products.

A possible alternative to industrial sugar, which is not exactly cheap, is coconut blossom sugar, which, despite its calories, keeps the blood sugar level more constant.

11. Check daily calorie intake

The Dash diet recommends a calorie intake between 1,500 and 2,300 kcal per day. If you want to lose weight, you should limit the value to 1,500 kcal per day. Of course, this is only a guideline and depends on the basal metabolic rate, age, body weight and size, muscular mass, gender, and health status. You can find a variety of calculators on the Internet to determine your calorie requirement (e.g., with Fit-for-Fun, Smart Calculator).

BEGINNING OF THE DASH DIET

Now that you are supplied with the necessary background information on the DASH diet let us see first what it entails. This meal plan is rich in vegetables, fruits, dairy products, whole grains, lean meats, poultry, fish, and legumes such as peas and beans. Additionally, it contains low fat from natural sources and high fiber from sweet potatoes, cabbage, and leafy vegetables. It adheres to the US guidelines about sodium and potassium content. It is a flexible eating plan designed to meet the needs of a variety of people and keep in mind their food preferences. There is a healthy alternative to almost any kind of food craving. It is what a typical DASH diet comprises. The table below shows the portions of food you can eat in a day based on the number of calories you want to take in.

TYPE OF FOOD	NUMBER OF SERVINGS (1600-3000 CALORIE PLAN)	NUMBER OF SERVINGS (1500-2000 CALORIE PLAN)
WHOLE GRAINS OR MEALS MADE OUT OF WHOLE GRAINS	6-12	7-9
FRESH FRUITS (NOT FRUIT JUICE)	4-5	4-6
FARM FRESH VEGETABLES (TRY AVOIDING STORE-BOUGHT ONES)	4-6	4-6
DAIRY PRODUCTS (LOW FAT)	3-4	2-4
POULTRY, FISH ¿, LEAN MEATS	2-3	3-4
LEGUMES, SEEDS, AND NUTS	3-5	4-5
DESSERTS, NATURAL FATS	2-3	2

THE IMPORTANCE OF EXERCISE DURING DIET

Increasing how much physical activity you do is an extremely important part of any weight-loss program. It is essential for several health reasons.

BURNS CALORIES

Physical activity is fundamental to the Dash Diet for Weight Loss because it burns calories.

BOOSTS METABOLISM

The more muscle in our anatomies, the faster our metabolism and the more calories we burn. Once we grow old, we naturally begin to lose muscle tissue, which in turn causes our metabolism to decelerate.

A VICIOUS CYCLE OCCURS

The less muscle we have, the slower our metabolism is, and the slower our metabolism, the more likely it is that we will gain weight. Physical activity is the key to breaking this cycle. Regular physical activity means you build muscle, which in turn means your metabolism will speed up. The beauty of this is that more muscle speeds up our metabolism even when we are at rest, not just when we are working out.

INCREASES STRENGTH

It is crucial to maintain muscle strength. Even if we do not need strength to do heavy work, having strong muscles allows us to do even routine daily activities more easily. It also helps us avoid injuries.

IMPROVED FITNESS MEANS BETTER HEALTH

Being physically fit is good for you. Most of us know that. Sometimes it is surprising to learn just how good it is for us. Exercise is so powerful that people who start exercising improve their health even if they do not lose any weight.

Exercise:

- Reduces the threat of cardiovascular disease and stroke.
- Reduces the danger of developing diabetes.
- Reduces the risk of some types of cancer.
- Improves sexual function.
- Increases your possibility of living longer.
- Improves your mood.

WALKING

Walking has many health advantages and is a minimal impact

on aerobic fitness exercise. Of most types of exercise, walking may be the simplest, lowest, and many basic forms. Everybody knows how to walk, and walking requires no specialized training or specific gear.

There are benefits of walking:

- Lowering cholesterol
- Lowering blood pressure
- Losing weight
- Reducing the threat of diabetes
- Restricting a depressed mood
- Increasing strength

Walking is not a fitness with many threats of injury; however, it is crucial to consider it easy in your body when getting into any new workout program. Do not intend to walk five miles if you are just getting started. Be realistic. Focus on one mile or less for the first few tries, and slowly boost your distance and speed as the body becomes strong. A very important thing about walking is that it is free. You can do it outside your entryway. It is wonderful to hear your preferred music, an audiobook, or even a motivational program while walking. The new air and visual impressions are great for the soul.

ADDITIONAL LOW IMPACT AEROBIC FITNESS EXERCISE

When it is too cold to walk, you can find other light aerobic fitness exercise options that you could take part in. You might desire to buy a tai chi exercise video or join a program at your local community center.

Other light aerobic exercise programs and activities include cardio step exercise, stationary bicycling, or walking on a treadmill. These activities might have a cost involved and a small learning curve, but they are low impact and carry the same health benefits as walking. It is essential always to wear proper footwear when doing any exercise program and to stay adequately hydrated.

YOGA

Yoga includes a note aerobic fitness exercise which has many health advantages, such as:

- Increased flexibility
- Increased strength
- Balanced mood
- Lower blood pressure
- Weight management
- Reduced stress
- Increased concentration
- Reduced insomnia
- Increased cardiovascular capacity

It's important to understand yoga from a trained yoga instructor. Yoga is usually a minimal impact exercise; nonetheless, it does have certain risks involved. If you do not understand the correct body positioning when trying to accomplish a yoga pose, you can pull a muscle or otherwise injure yourself. Most gyms and community centers offer beginner yoga classes for a small fee in a friendly environment.

SWIMMING

Swimming and water aerobatics tend to be called ideal exercises. It is a minimal impact on aerobic fitness exercise that is done in a weightless environment. The health benefit of swimming is that it acts like walking but with the added advantage of having zero effect on your body because of the weightlessness experienced in the water. This makes swimming and water exercise ideal for older adults and folks with injuries or arthritis.

The downside of swimming is the fact that it can require someone to learn how to swim. Water aerobics takes a pool. Many health clubs have indoor, heated pools and provide swimming classes and aerobic water classes.

The Dash diet involves an exercise component. Exercise is essential in reducing weight and decreasing blood pressure. The advantages cannot be emphasized enough.

Select a program or several programs that can best suit your way of life and do at least 20 minutes of exercise 3 times a week.

After a month, increase this to 30-45 minutes, up to 5 times a week. You will not only look better and have lower blood pressure, but you will also FEEL much better as well.

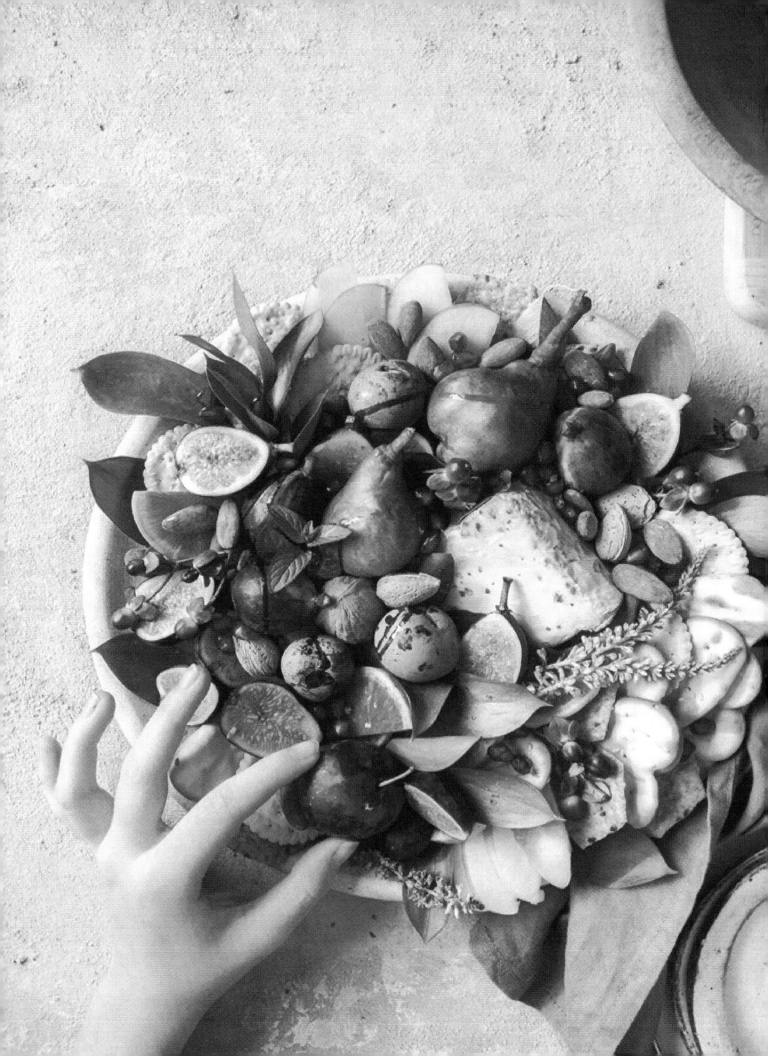

CHAPTER 2
BENEFITS OF THE DASH DIET

Although you're likely to go for the DASH diet because of a slimmer waist and better health, there are more reasons to consider the DASH diet. They include the following:

CONTROLLED BLOOD PRESSURE

This is the main benefit of the DASH diet and the reason why nutritionists and physicians recommend it. Following DASH lets you keep your blood pressure in check. This diet is ideal for anyone who is taking medication to control blood pressure as well as those with prehypertension symptoms and are looking for better ways of managing these symptoms. DASH is specially designed to help tame blood pressure and has been scientifically proven to work.

HEALTHY EATING

Let's face it. One of the reasons most people experience high blood pressure is that being overweight or obese is associated with poor eating choices. Following the DASH diet helps you make a lifestyle change to healthy eating. Thus, you will be spending more time in the kitchen preparing fresh food instead of grabbing processed food on the go. You will also enjoy your meal times because your plate will be filled with more nutritious foods. DASH also stretches you a little to try out new vegetables and fruits and experiment with various seasonings that are salt-free to create meals that you will enjoy.

REDUCED RISK OF OSTEOPOROSIS

The majority of dietary approaches to preventing and treating osteoporosis include increasing your intake of calcium and vitamin D found in abundance in foods recommended for the DASH diet. This reduced sodium intake is proof that the DASH diet is quite beneficial for bone health. Some studies found a notable decline in bone turnover for people who followed the DASH diet. When sustained over a longer period, the DASH diet is instrumental in improving bone mineral status. Other nutrients that are in abundance in the DASH diet and are excellent at promoting bone health over time include vitamin C, antioxidants, magnesium, and polyphenols.

HEALTHY CHOLESTEROL LEVELS

Since most of the fruits, beans, nuts, whole grains, and vegetables recommended under the DASH diet have high fiber content, you can eat them alongside fish and lean meat while limiting your intake of refined carbohydrates and sweets. This goes a long way in improving your cholesterol levels.

BETTER WEIGHT MANAGEMENT

The DASH diet is a perfect option when you want to maintain a healthy weight or are keen on losing weight. You can follow a version of the DASH diet that is tailored to help you achieve weight loss goals, after which you can stick to a higher calorie count to maintain your ideal weight. This means you won't have to worry about gaining weight again. The DASH diet provides an abundance of proteins without including too many carbohydrates. Thus, you will be able to build muscle as well as boost your metabolism without feeling heavy. Even better, this is not a short-term change but a lifestyle.

HEALTHIER KIDNEYS

The DASH diet lowers the risk for kidney stones and kidney disease because of the abundance of magnesium, potassium, calcium, and fiber present in the foods encouraged. The focus on reducing sodium intake is also an advantage if you face the risk of developing kidney disease. Even then, the DASH diet should be restricted to patients who have chronic kidney disease and those undergoing dialysis without the close guidance of qualified health care professionals.

EASY TO MAINTAIN

The DASH diet is designed around readily available foods, making it easier to follow and maintain. Apart from comprising foods that leave you feeling satiated for most of the day, you can eat two or three snacks per day. When you commit to this diet, you can be sure to enjoy long-term changes in your lifestyle that are a plus for your overall wellness and health. You can even follow the DASH even when you're eating out at a restaurant because all you need to do is beware of those foods that are likely to jeopardize your efforts. Besides, there are many ways of making this diet work for you.

PREVENTS DIABETES

The DASH diet effectively prevents insulin resistance that has been linked to cardiovascular risks and high blood pressure. By managing your sodium intake, maintaining a healthy weight, and eating more potassium and fiber, this eating plan helps delay or avoid the onset of diabetes if you're predisposed to the disease. Studies have further shown that the impact is even better when you implement the DASH diet as a component of a comprehensive healthy lifestyle that includes exercise, diet, and weight control.

DECREASED RISK OF CERTAIN CANCERS

Researchers have studied the relationship between the DASH diet and certain types of cancers and found a positive association related to reducing salt intake and monitoring dietary fat consumption. The diet is also low in red, which is linked to cancer of the rectum, colon, esophagus, lung, stomach, kidney, and prostate. Eating plenty of fresh produce helps prevent various cancers while emphasizing dairy products low in fat contributes to a drop in the risk of colon cancer.

BETTER MENTAL HEALTH

The DASH diet will boost your mood while decreasing symptoms of mental health disorders like anxiety or depression. This is associated with various lifestyle changes that include avoiding cigarettes, moderating alcohol consumption, and exercising regularly. Moreover, the inclusion of nutrient-rich foods in the diet also helps in balancing out hormones and chemicals in the brain and body, thus contributing to improved mental health and overall well-being.

YOU FEEL LESS HUNGRY

By consuming high in protein and high fiber foods, the DASH diet will leave no room for cravings for fast foods. Instead, you tend to feel more satiated throughout the day and only look forward to the next nutritious and filling meal. However, you can always identify some DASH-friendly snacks if you feel you need to snack. Cutting on carbs and eating low-fat diets can leave you feeling restricted and hungry; however, the DASH diet is easier to stick to because it keeps you satisfied.

HEALTHY LIFESTYLE

The DASH plan is more than the diet; it's more about being able to take control of your health and wellness in manageable ways. Thus, by balancing between healthy living, exercise, and nutrition, you can be sure to see a broader range of valuable benefits in addition to the wellness that you will experience with the DASH diet plan.

ANTI-AGING PROPERTIES

Many people who follow the DASH diet have attested that this diet helps avoid some effects of aging so that they keep them feeling and looking younger. Increasing your consumption of fresh vegetables and fruits that are full of antioxidants will rejuvenate your hair and skin, revitalize and strengthen your joints, muscles, and bones, help you lose weight, and leave you feeling healthier.

IMPROVED COGNITIVE FUNCTION

According to research, the DASH diet will help keep your brain sharp and avoid memory loss, thus significantly slowing your mental decline rate. Besides, high fiber and low-fat eating can promote lower blood pressure, which is usually a risk factor in developing degenerative conditions like dementia and Alzheimer's disease. Some of the best foods that help curb mental decline included in the DASH diet include whole grains, vegetables, low-fat dairy, legumes, and nuts.

REDUCED RISK OF DEVELOPING HEART DISEASE

The ability of the DASH diet to keep your blood pressure in check is instrumental in strengthening the body's resistance to heart disease. According to a 2010 study, DASH can substantially lower the risk of heart disease. This is particularly great given the persistent and enormous burden of coronary heart disease. This finding is attributed to the fact that lowered blood pressure lets the heart function efficiently and effectively. Moreover, it can also be beneficial for those not struggling with hypertension but are keen on preventing the onset of heart disease.

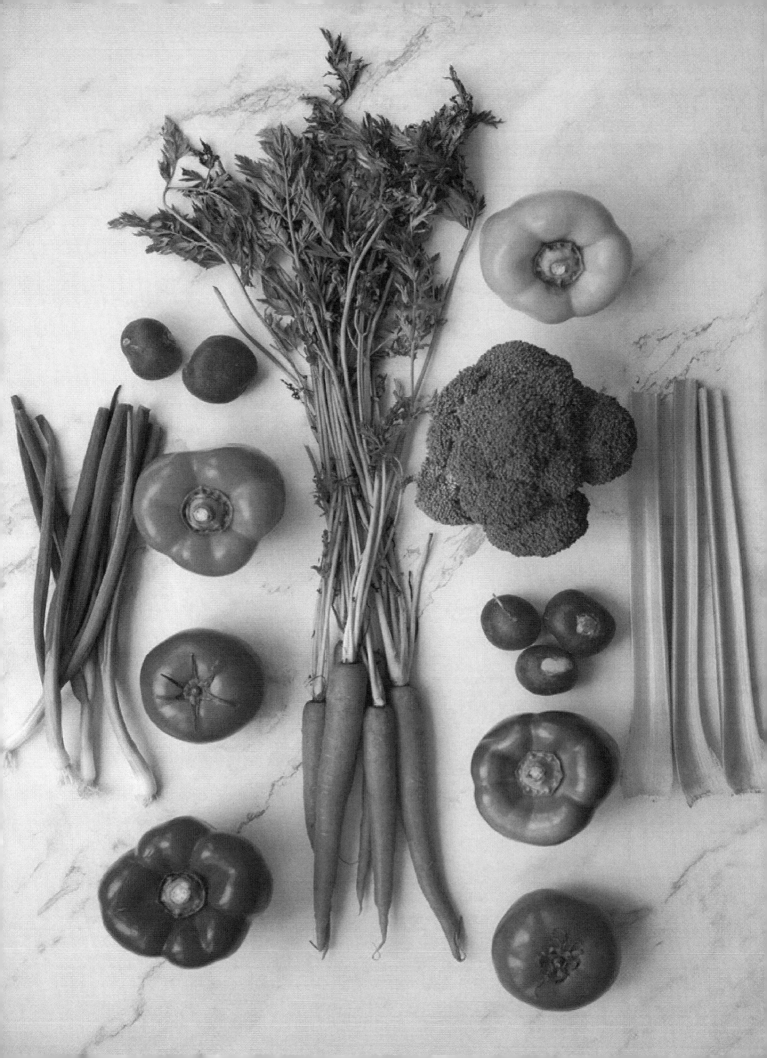

CHAPTER 3
28-DAY MEAL PLAN

WEEK 1

DAY	BREAKFAST	LUNCH	DINNER
1	AVOCADO CUP WITH EGG	GARLIC MUSHROOM CHICKEN	EASY BEEF BRISKET
2	GREEK YOGURT OAT PANCAKES	CHICKEN WRAP	BAKED FISH SERVED WITH VEGETABLES
3	BROWN SUGAR CINNAMON OATMEAL	TUNA SANDWICH	PAELLA WITH CHICKEN, LEEKS, AND TARRAGON
4	ALMOND BUTTER-BANANA SMOOTHIE	TOFU & GREEN BEAN STIR-FRY	SALSA CHICKEN CHILI
5	SAVORY YOGURT BOWLS	ITALIAN STUFFED PORTOBELLO MUSHROOM BURGERS	CHICKEN WITH MUSHROOMS
6	OATMEAL BANANA PANCAKES WITH WALNUTS	CURRY VEGETABLE NOODLES WITH CHICKEN	OLIVE CAPERS CHICKEN
7	SWEET BERRIES PANCAKE	BLACK BEAN STEW WITH CORNBREAD	SOUTHWESTERN CHICKEN AND PASTA

WEEK 2

DAY	BREAKFAST	LUNCH	DINNER
1	CARROT MUFFINS	EGGPLANT PARMESAN STACKS	BEEF STEW WITH FENNEL AND SHALLOTS
2	PUMPKIN MUFFINS	DILL AND LEMON COD PACKETS	STUFFED CHICKEN BREASTS
3	APPLE PANCAKES	SALMON WRAP	HONEY CRUSTED CHICKEN
4	STRAWBERRY SANDWICH	SWEET POTATOES AND ZUCCHINI SOUP	PORK AND ROASTED TOMATOES MIX
5	SCRAMBLED EGG AND VEGGIE BREAKFAST QUESADILLAS	CHICKPEA CAULIFLOWER TIKKA MASALA	EASY SHRIMP
6	ENERGY SUNRISE MUFFINS	MEXICAN-STYLE POTATO CASSEROLE	BASIL HALIBUT
7	CREAMY OATS & BLUEBERRY SMOOTHIE	DILL CHICKEN SALAD	WHITE BEANS WITH SPINACH AND PAN-ROASTED TOMATOES

WEEK 3

DAY	BREAKFAST	LUNCH	DINNER
1	SPINACH, EGG, AND CHEESE BREAKFAST QUESADILLAS	SWEET AND SOUR CHICKEN WHIT NOODLES AND VEGETABLE	LEEK & CAULIFLOWER SOUP
2	BLUEBERRY WAFFLES	STEAMED SALMON TERIYAKI	PORK MEDALLIONS WITH FIVE SPICE POWDER
3	SUPER-SIMPLE GRANOLA	LIGHT BALSAMIC SALAD	MUSTARD CHICKEN TENDERS
4	BREAKFAST BANANA SPLIT	LEMONGRASS AND CHICKEN SOUP	SPICY COD
5	BREAKFAST FRUITS BOWLS	FRUITED QUINOA SALAD	GRILLED PORK FAJITAS
6	EASY VEGGIE MUFFINS	EASY LUNCH SALMON STEAKS	PROVENCE PORK MEDALLIONS
7	MUSHROOMS AND CHEESE OMELET	WHITE CHICKEN CHILI	COCONUT SHRIMP

WEEK 4

DAY	BREAKFAST	LUNCH	DINNER
1	APPLE QUINOA MUFFINS	EASY STEAMED ALASKAN COD	SIMPLE BEEF BRISKET AND TOMATO SOUP
2	STEEL CUT OAT BLUEBERRY PANCAKES	PORK AND DATES SAUCE	FISH IN A VEGETABLE PATCH
3	PINEAPPLE OATMEAL	SWEET POTATO-TURKEY MEATLOAF	STEAMED BLUE CRABS
4	BANANA & CINNAMON OATMEAL	TURKEY WRAP	ASIAN SALMON
5	ZUCCHINI PANCAKES	WHITE BEANS STEW	GARLIC PEPPER CHICKEN
6	CARROT CAKE OVERNIGHT OATS	SPICY TOFU BURRITO BOWLS WITH CILANTRO AVOCADO SAUCE	BAKED CHICKEN
7	EGG WHITE BREAKFAST MIX	CHICKEN WITH POTATOES OLIVES & SPROUTS	GINGER SESAME SALMON

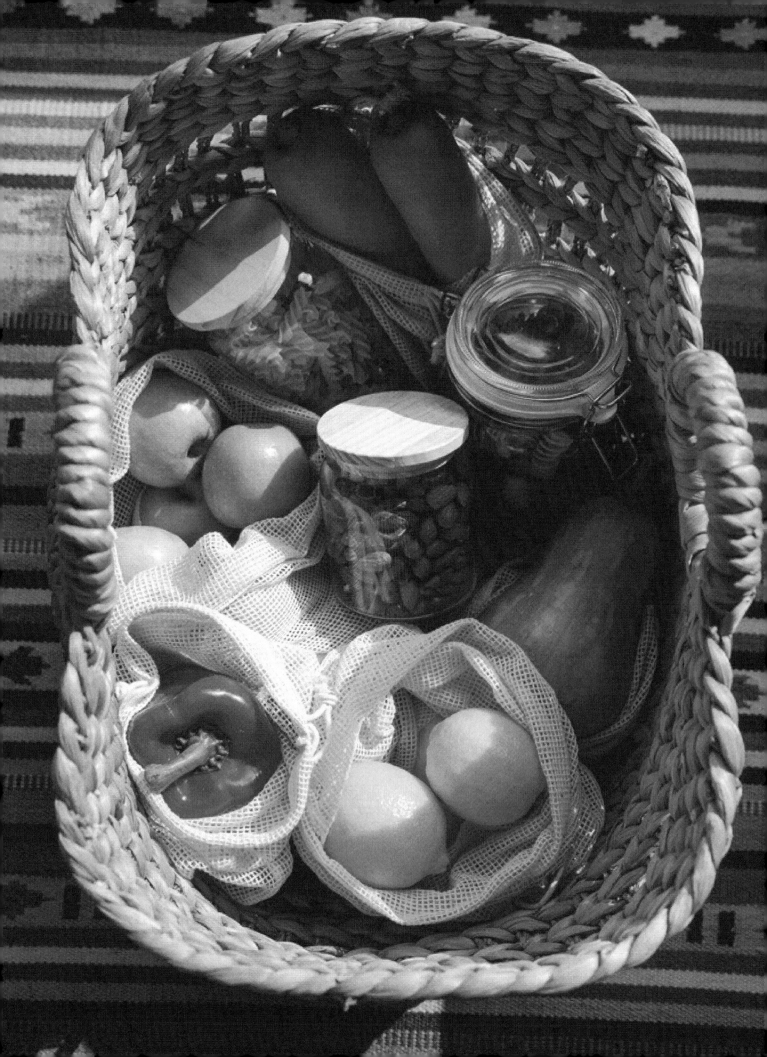

CHAPTER 4

SHOPPING LIST

Here you find a list of the foods you should put in your shopping cart to succeed while following the DASH Diet. You'll find many tasty and varied kinds of foods. Thus meal preparations won't be tedious, and you can still enjoy cooking and preparing healthy and delicious meals.

WEEK 1

PARMESAN CHEESE	1 BLOCK		LEMON	3 PCS
SCALLION	½ LB		COD FILLET	½ LB
AVOCADO	5		ZUCCHINI	¼ LB
EGG	1 DOZEN		PARSLEY	1 BUNCH
CHICKEN	5 LB		BROWN SUGAR	¼ LB
GARLIC	¼ LB		FAT MILK	½ GAL
ONION	¼ LB		OATS	1 PACK
MUSHROOM	1 CAN		TUNA	¼ LB
BEEF	2 LB		LETTUCE	1 HEAD
TOMATOES	¼ LB		PEAS	1/8 LB
RED PEPPER	2 PCS		MOZZARELLA CHEESE	1 LB
ALMOND BUTTER	1 PACKED		PANCAKE MIX	1 PACK
TOFU	2 BLOCKS		STRAWBERRY	¼ LB
CUCUMBER	2 PCS		BLUEBERRY	¼ LB
KALAMATA OLIVES	1 CAN		RIGATONI	1 PACK
GREEK YOGURT	16 OZ		TOMATO SAUCE	2 PACKS
BREAD CRUMBS	1 PACK		SALSA	1 PACKAGE
ARUGULA	1 BUNCH		BROWN RICE	1 PACKAGE
BANANA	6 PCS			

DASH DIET 2022

WEEK 2

EGG	1 DOZEN		SHRIMP	2 LB
COD FILLET	½ LB		SALMON	1 LB
			GARLIC	¼ LB
PORK	2 LB		ONION	¼ LB
CHICKEN	5 LB		CARROT	½ LB
MUSHROOM	1 CAN		GINGER	3
BEEF	2 LB		PECAN	¼ LB
TOMATOES	¼ LB		EGGPLANT	3
BANANA	3 PCS		MOZZARELLA CHEESE	1 BLOCK
LEMON	3 PCS		PARMESAN CHEESE	1 BLOCK
ZUCCHINI	¼ LB			
PARSLEY	1 BUNCH		SHALLOT	½ LB
BROWN SUGAR	¼ LB		FENNEL BULB	½ LB
FAT MILK	½ GAL		BAY LEAF	4
PEAS	1/8 LB		POTATOES	½ LB
RED PEPPER	2 PCS		WALNUT	1 PACK
ALMOND BUTTER	1 PACKED		TORTILLA WRAP	1 PACK
SPINACH	1 BUNCH		STRAWBERRIES	½ LB
APPLE	3		COCONUT MILK	1 CAN
CRANBERRY	½ LB		CAULIFLOWER	2
BROWN RICE	1 PACK		RAISINS	1 PACK
INSTANT NOODLES	1		ORANGE	2

WEEK 3

EGG	1/2 DOZEN	SPINACH	1 BUNCH
PORK	2 LB	APPLE	3 PCS
CHICKEN	5 LB	CRANBERRY	½ LB
WHOLE-WHEAT SPAGHETTI	1/2 LB	CARROT	½ LB
GARLIC	¼ LB	GINGER	3 PCS
ONION	¼ LB	MOZZARELLA CHEESE	1 BLOCK
MUSHROOM	1 CAN	PARMESAN CHEESE	1 BLOCK
TOMATOES	¼ LB	GARLIC	½ LB
BANANA	3 PCS	ONION	½ LB
LEMON	3 PCS	POTATOES	½ LB
PARSLEY	1 BUNCH	WALNUT	1 PACK
BROWN SUGAR	¼ LB	TORTILLA WRAP	1 PACK
RED PEPPER	2 PCS	STRAWBERRIES	½ LB
ALMOND BUTTER	1 PACKED	BLUEBERRIES	½ LB
COCONUT MILK	1 CAN	MANGO	2 PCS
CAULIFLOWER	2 PCS	BROCCOLI	2 PCS
BROWN RICE	1 PACK	GREEN PEPPER	2 PCS
RAISINS	1 PACK	RED PEPPER	2 PCS
ORANGE	2 PCS	REDUCED-FAT MONTEREY JACK CHEESE	1 BLOCK
PINEAPPLE	1 PCS		

DASH DIET 2022
WEEK 4

QUINOA	1 PACK		HALIBUT FILLET	1 LB
EGG	1 DOZEN		CRAB	1 LB
COD FILLET	½ LB		GARLIC	¼ LB
PORK	2 LB		ONION	¼ LB
CHICKEN	4 LBS.		TOMATOES	¼ LB
BEEF	2 ½ LB		BANANA	3 PCS
TURKEY BREAST	1 LB		LEMON	3 PCS
SALMON FILLET	1 LB		ZUCCHINI	1/2 LB
BROWN SUGAR	¼ LB		TORTILLA WRAP	1 PACK
ALMOND MILK	½ GAL		COCONUT MILK	1 CAN
RED PEPPER	2 PCS		BROWN RICE	1 PACK
SPINACH	1 BUNCH		RAISINS	1 PACK
APPLE	3		ORANGE	2
CARROT	½ LB		GREEK YOGURT	16 OZ
GINGER	3		DATES	1/8 LB
FETA CHEESE	1 BLOCK		PINEAPPLE	1
PARMESAN CHEESE	1 BLOCK		KETCHUP	1
POTATOES	½ LB		BEER	1
WALNUT	1 PACK		VINEGAR	1

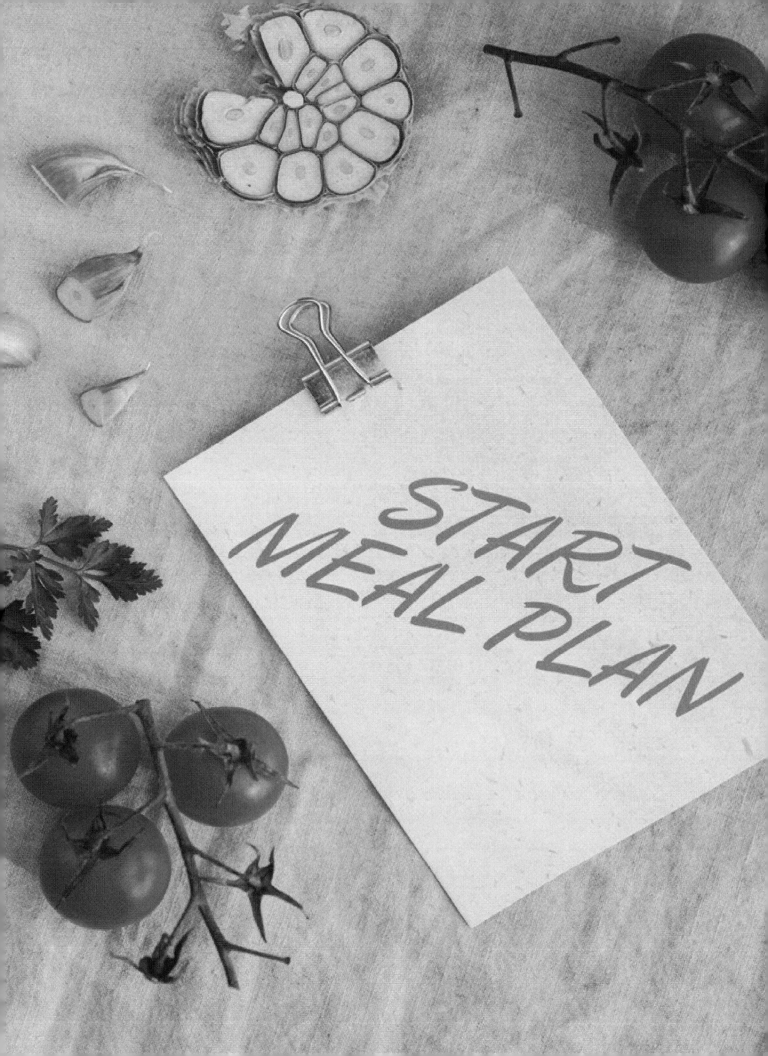

CHAPTER 5

MEAL PLAN WEEK 1

DASH DIET 2022

DAY 1

BREAKFAST

AVOCADO CUP WITH EGG

INGREDIENTS

- 4 teaspoons of parmesan cheese
- 4 dashes of pepper
- 4 dashes of paprika
- 2 ripe avocados
- 4 medium eggs

NUTRITIONAL FACTS:

Calories: 206, Fat: 15.4 g, Carbs: 11.3 g, Protein: 8.5 g, Sugars; 0.4 g, Sodium: 21 mg

COOKING: 0'

PREPARATION: 5'

SERVES: 4

DIRECTIONS

1. Preheat oven to 375 °F. Slice the avocadoes in half and discard the seed. Slice the rounded portions of the avocado to make it level and sit well on a baking sheet.

2. Place the avocadoes on a baking sheet and crack one egg in each hole of the avocado. Season each egg evenly with pepper and paprika. Bake within 25 minutes or until eggs are cooked to your liking. Serve with a sprinkle of parmesan.

LUNCH

GARLIC MUSHROOM CHICKEN

INGREDIENTS

- 4 chicken breasts, boneless and skinless
- 3 garlic cloves, minced
- 1 onion, chopped
- 2 cups of mushrooms, sliced
- 1 tablespoon of olive oil
- ½ cup of chicken stock
- ¼ teaspoon of pepper
- ½ teaspoon of salt

NUTRITIONAL FACTS:

Calories: 331, Fat: 14.5 g, Protein: 43.9 g, Carbs: 4.6 g, Sodium 420 mg

COOKING: 15'

PREPARATION: 15'

SERVES: 4

DIRECTIONS

1. Season the chicken with pepper and salt. Warm the oil in a pan on medium heat, then put the seasoned chicken in the pan and cook for 5-6 minutes on each side. Remove and place on a plate.

2. Add the onion and mushrooms to the pan and sauté until tender, about 2-3 minutes. Add the garlic and sauté for a minute. Add the stock and bring to boil. Stir well and cook for 1-2 minutes. Pour over chicken and serve.

DINNER

EASY BEEF BRISKET

INGREDIENTS

- 1 teaspoon of thyme
- 4 cloves of garlic, peeled & smashed
- 1 ½ cups of onion, chopped
- 2 ½ lbs. of beef brisket, chopped
- 1 tablespoon of olive oil
- ¼ teaspoon of Black Pepper
- 14.5 ounces of tomatoes & liquid, Canned
- ¼ cup of red wine vinegar
- 1 cup of beef stock, low sodium

NUTRITIONAL FACTS:

Calories: 299, Protein: 10.2 g, Fat: 9 g
Carbs: 21.4 g, Sodium: 372 mg,
Cholesterol: 101 mg

COOKING: 1H 10'

PREPARATION: 2H

SERVES: 4

DIRECTIONS

1. Turn the oven to 350 °F, and then grease a Dutch oven using a tablespoon of oil. Place it over medium heat.

2. Add your pepper and brisket. Cook until it browns, and then place your brisket on a plate.

3. Put your onions in the pot, and cook until golden brown. Stir in your garlic and thyme, cooking for another full minute before adding the stock, vinegar, and tomatoes.

4. Cook until it comes to a boil, and then add in your brisket again.

5. Reduce to a simmer, and cook for 3 hours in the oven until tender.

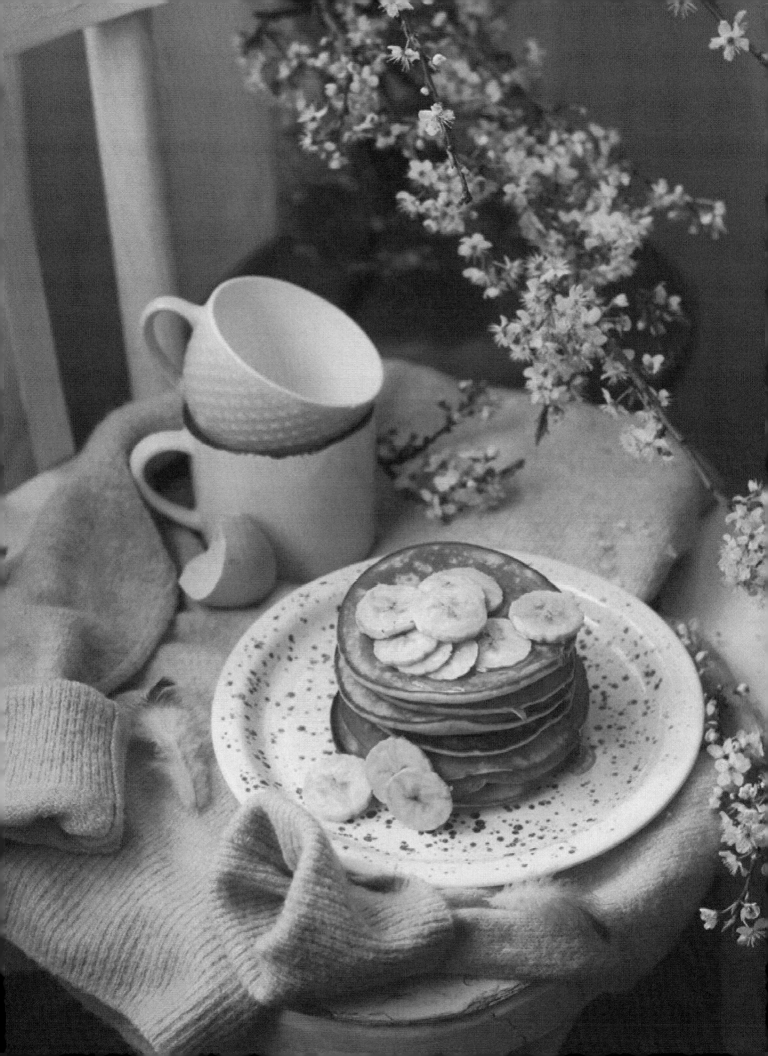

DAY 2

DASH DIET 2022

BREAKFAST

GREEK YOGURT OAT PANCAKES

INGREDIENTS

- 6 egg whites
  (or ¾ cup of liquid egg whites)
- 1 cup of rolled oats
- 1 cup of plain nonfat Greek yogurt
- 1 medium banana, peeled and sliced
- 1 teaspoon of ground cinnamon
- 1 teaspoon of baking powder

NUTRITIONAL FACTS:

Calories: 318, Fat: 4 g, Sodium: 467 mg, Potassium: 634 mg, Carbs: 47 g, Fiber: 6 g, Sugars: 13 g, Protein: 28 g

COOKING: 10'

PREPARATION: 15'

SERVES: 2

DIRECTIONS

1. Blend all of the listed ingredients using a blender. Warm a griddle over medium heat. Spray the skillet with nonstick cooking spray.

2. Put 1/3 cup of the mixture or batter onto the griddle. Allow to cook and flip when bubbles on the top burst, about 5 minutes. Cook again within a minute until golden brown. Repeat with the remaining batter. Divide between two serving plates and enjoy.

LUNCH

CHICKEN WRAP

INGREDIENTS

- 1 tablespoon of extra-virgin olive oil
- Lemon juice of 2 lemons, divided into 3 parts
- 2 cloves of garlic, minced
- 1 lb. of boneless skinless chicken breasts
- ½ cup of non-fat plain Greek yogurt
- ½ teaspoon of paprika
- Pinch of salt and pepper
- Hot sauce to taste
- Pita bread
- Tomato slice

NUTRITIONAL FACTS:

Calories: 348, Carbs: 8.7 g, Proteins: 56 g, Fat: 10.2 g, Sodium: 198 mg

COOKING: 15'

PREPARATION: 15'

SERVES: 2

DIRECTIONS

1. Whisk 1 tablespoon of olive oil, juice of 2 lemons, garlic, salt, and pepper for the marinade in a bowl. Add the chicken breasts to the marinade and place it into a large Ziploc. Let marinate for 30 mins to 4 hours.

2. Mix the yogurt, hot sauce, and the remaining lemon juice season with paprika and a pinch of salt and pepper for the yogurt sauce.

3. Warm the skillet over medium heat and coat it with oil. Add the chicken breast and cook until golden brown and cook about 8 minutes per side. Remove from pan and let it rest for a few minutes, then slice.

4. To a piece of pita bread, add lettuce, tomato, and chicken slices. Drizzle with the prepared spicy yogurt sauce. Serve and enjoy!

DINNER

BAKED FISH SERVED WITH VEGETABLES

INGREDIENTS

- 4 haddock or cod fillets, skinless
- 2 zucchinis, sliced into thick pieces
- 2 red onions, sliced into thick pieces
- 3 large tomatoes, cut into wedges
- ¼ cup of black olives pitted
- ¼ cup of flavorless oil (olive, canola, or sunflower)
- 1 tablespoon of lemon juice
- 1 tablespoon of Dijon mustard
- 2 garlic cloves, minced
- Salt and pepper to season
- ½ cup of chopped parsley

NUTRITIONAL FACTS:

Calories : 91, Protein: 18.7 g, Carbs: 41 g, Fat: 7.6 g, Sodium: 199 mg

COOKING: 30'

PREPARATION: 15'

SERVES: 4

DIRECTIONS

1. Warm the oven to 400 °F. In a large baking dish, drizzle some oil over the bottom. Place the fish in the middle. Surround the fish with zucchini, tomato, onion, and olives. Drizzle more oil over the vegetables and fish—season with salt and pepper.

2. Place the baking dish in the oven. Now bake within 30 minutes, or until the fish is flaky and vegetables are tender. In another bowl, whisk the lemon juice, garlic, mustard, and remaining oil. Set aside.

3. Split the cooked vegetables onto plates, then top with the fish. Drizzle the dressing over the vegetables, fish. Garnish with parsley.

DASH DIET 2022

DAY 3

BREAKFAST

BROWN SUGAR CINNAMON OATMEAL

INGREDIENTS

- ½ teaspoon of ground cinnamon
- 1 ½ teaspoon of pure vanilla extract
- ¼ cup of light brown sugar
- 2 cups of low-fat milk
- 1 1/3 cup of quick oats

NUTRITIONAL FACTS:

Calories: 208, Fat: 3 g, Carbs: 38 g
Protein: 8 g, Sugars: 15 g, Sodium: 33 mg

COOKING: 3'

PREPARATION: 1'

SERVES: 4

DIRECTIONS

1. Put the milk plus vanilla into a medium saucepan and boil over medium-high heat.
2. Lower the heat to medium once it boils. Mix in oats, brown sugar, plus cinnamon, and cook, stirring for 2–3 minutes. Serve immediately.

LUNCH

TUNA SANDWICH

INGREDIENTS

- 2 slices of whole-grain bread
- 1 can (6-ounces) of low sodium tuna in water, in its juice
- 2 teaspoons of Yogurt (1.5% fat) or low-fat mayonnaise
- 1 medium tomato, diced
- ½ small sweet onion, finely diced
- Lettuce leaves

NUTRITIONAL FACTS:

Calories: 235, Fat: 3 g, Protein: 27.8 g, Sodium: 350 mg, Carbs: 25.9 g

COOKING: 0'

PREPARATION: 15'

SERVES: 1

DIRECTIONS

1. Toast the whole grain bread slices. Mix the tuna, yogurt, or mayonnaise, diced tomato, and onion. Cover a toasted bread with lettuce leaves and spread the tuna mixture on the sandwich. Spread the tuna mixture on toasted bread with lettuce leaves. Place another disc as a cover on top. Enjoy the sandwich.

DINNER

PAELLA WITH CHICKEN, LEEKS, AND TARRAGON

INGREDIENTS

- 1 teaspoon of extra-virgin olive oil
- 1 small onion, sliced
- 2 leeks (whites only), thinly sliced
- 3 garlic cloves, minced
- 1-pound of boneless, skinless chicken breast, cut into strips 1/2-inch-wide and 2 inches long
- 2 large tomatoes, chopped
- 1 red pepper, sliced
- 2/3 cup of long-grain brown rice
- 1 teaspoon of tarragon, or to taste
- 2 cups of fat-free, unsalted chicken broth
- 1 cup of frozen peas
- ¼ cup of chopped fresh parsley
- 1 lemon, cut into 4 wedges

NUTRITIONAL FACTS:

Calories: 388 , Fat: 15.2 g, Sodium: 572 mg, Carbs: 5.4 g, Protein: 27 g

COOKING: 20'

PREPARATION: 10'

SERVES: 2

DIRECTIONS

1. Preheat a nonstick pan with olive oil over medium heat. Toss in leeks, onions, chicken strips, and garlic. Sauté for 5 minutes. Stir in red pepper slices and tomatoes. Stir and cook for 5 minutes.

2. Add the tarragon, broth, and rice. Let it boil, then reduce the heat to a simmer. Continue cooking for 10 minutes, then add peas and continue cooking until the liquid is thoroughly cooked. Garnish with parsley and lemon. Serve.

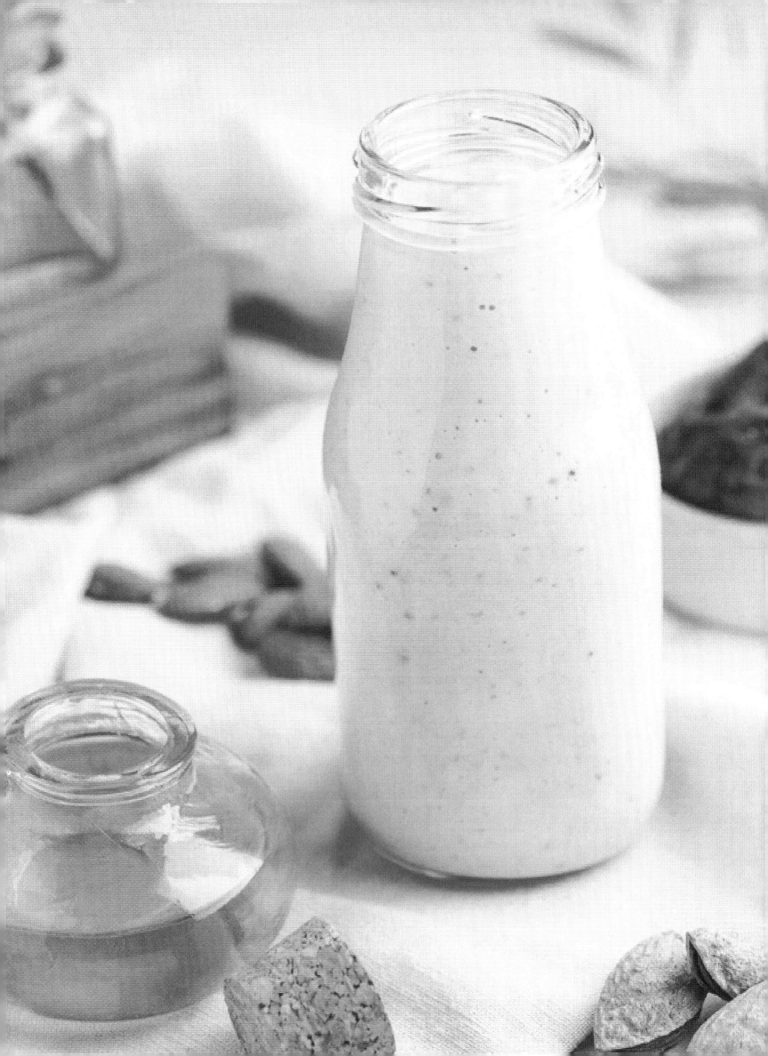

DAY 4

BREAKFAST

ALMOND BUTTER-BANANA SMOOTHIE

INGREDIENTS

- 1 tablespoon of almond butter
- ½ cup of ice cubes
- 1 peeled and a frozen medium banana
- 1 cup of fat-free milk

NUTRITIONAL FACTS:

Calories: 293, Fat: 9.8 g,
Carbs: 42.5 g, Protein: 13.5 g,
Sugars: 12 g, Sodium: 40 mg

COOKING: 0'

PREPARATION: 5'

SERVES: 1

DIRECTIONS

1. Blend all the listed ingredients above in a powerful blender until smooth and creamy. Serve and enjoy.

LUNCH

TOFU & GREEN BEAN STIR-FRY

INGREDIENTS

- 1 (14-ounces) package of extra-firm tofu
- 12 tablespoons of canola oil
- 1-pound of green beans, chopped
- 2 carrots, peeled and thinly sliced
- ½ cup of Stir-Fry Sauce or store-bought lower-sodium stir-fry sauce
- 2 cups of fluffy brown rice
- 2 scallions, thinly sliced
- 2 tablespoons of sesame seeds

NUTRITIONAL FACTS:

Calories: 380, Fat: 15 g, Sodium: 440 mg, Potassium: 454 mg, Carbs: 45 g, Protein: 16 g

COOKING: 20'

PREPARATION: 15'

SERVES: 4

DIRECTIONS

1. Put the tofu on your plate lined with a kitchen towel, put a separate kitchen towel over the tofu, and place a heavy pot on top, changing towels every time they become soaked. Let sit within 15 minutes to remove the moisture. Cut the tofu into 1-inch cubes.

2. Heat the canola oil in a large wok or skillet to medium-high heat. Add the tofu cubes and cook, flipping every 1 to 2 minutes, so all sides become browned. Remove from the skillet and place the green beans and carrots in the hot oil. Stir-fry for 4 to 5 minutes, occasionally tossing, until crisp and slightly tender.

3. While the vegetables are cooking, prepare the Stir-Fry Sauce (if using homemade). Place the tofu back in the skillet. Put the sauce over the tofu and vegetables and let simmer for 2 to 3 minutes. Serve over rice, then top with scallions and sesame seeds.

DINNER

SALSA CHICKEN CHILI

INGREDIENTS

- 2 ½ lbs. of chicken breasts, skinless and boneless
- 1/2 teaspoon of cumin powder
- 3 garlic cloves, minced
- 1 onion, diced
- 16 ounces of hot salsa
- 1 teaspoon of oregano
- 1 tablespoon of olive oil

NUTRITIONAL FACTS:

Calories: 308, Fat: 12.4 g, Protein: 42.1 g, Carbs: 5.4 g, Sodium 656 mg

COOKING: 20'

PREPARATION: 15'

SERVES: 8

DIRECTIONS

1. Add oil into the instant pot and set the pot on sauté mode. Add onion to the pot and sauté until softened, about 3 minutes. Add garlic and sauté for a minute. Add oregano and cumin and sauté for a minute. Add half salsa and stir well. Place chicken and pour remaining salsa over chicken.

2. Seal pot with the lid and select manual, and set timer for 10 minutes. Remove chicken and shred. Move it back to the pot, then stir well to combine. Serve and enjoy.

DASH DIET 2022

DAY 5

BREAKFAST

SAVORY YOGURT BOWLS

INGREDIENTS

- 1 medium cucumber, diced
- ½ cup of pitted Kalamata olives halved
- 2 tablespoons of fresh lemon juice
- 1 tablespoon of extra-virgin olive oil
- 1 teaspoon of dried oregano
- ¼ teaspoon of freshly ground black pepper
- 2 cups of nonfat plain Greek yogurt
- ½ cup of slivered almonds

NUTRITIONAL FACTS:

Calories: 240, Fat: 16 g, Carbs: 10 g, Protein: 16 g, Potassium: 353 mg, Sodium: 350 mg

COOKING: 0'

PREPARATION: 15'

SERVES: 4

DIRECTIONS

1. Mix the cucumber, olives, lemon juice, oil, oregano, and pepper in a small bowl. Divide the yogurt evenly among 4 storage containers. Top with the cucumber-olive mix and almonds.

LUNCH

ITALIAN STUFFED PORTOBELLO MUSHROOM BURGERS

INGREDIENTS

- 1 tablespoon of olive oil
- 4 large portobello mushrooms, washed and dried
- ½ yellow onion, peeled and diced
- 4 garlic cloves, peeled and minced
- 1 can of cannellini beans, drained
- ½ cup of fresh basil leaves, torn
- ½ cup of panko bread crumbs
- 1/8 teaspoon of kosher or sea salt
- ¼ teaspoon of ground black pepper
- 1 cup of lower-sodium marinara, divided
- ½ cup of shredded mozzarella cheese
- 4 whole-wheat buns, toasted
- 1 cup of fresh arugula

NUTRITIONAL FACTS:

Calories: 407, Fat: 9 g, Sodium: 575 mg, Carbs: 63 g, Protein: 25 g

COOKING: 25'

PREPARATION: 15'

SERVES: 4

DIRECTIONS

1. Heat the olive oil in a large skillet to medium-high heat. Sear the mushrooms for 4 to 5 minutes per side, until slightly soft. Place on a baking sheet. Preheat the oven to low heat.

2. Put the onion in the skillet and cook for 4 to 5 minutes, until slightly soft. Mix in the garlic, then cook within 30 to 60 seconds. Move the onions plus garlic to a bowl. Add the cannellini beans and smash with the back of a fork to form a chunky paste. Stir in the basil, bread crumbs, salt, black pepper, and half of the marinara. Cook for 5 minutes.

3. Remove the bean mixture from the stove and divide it among the mushroom caps. Spoon the remaining marinara over the stuffed mushrooms and top each with mozzarella cheese. Broil within 3 to 4 minutes, until the cheese is melted and bubbly. Transfer the burgers to the toasted whole-wheat buns and top with the arugula.

DINNER

CHICKEN WITH MUSHROOMS

INGREDIENTS

- 2 chicken breasts, skinless and boneless
- 1 cup of mushrooms, sliced
- 1 onion, sliced
- 1 cup of chicken stock
- ½ teaspoon of thyme, dried
- Pepper
- Salt

NUTRITIONAL FACTS:

Calories: 313, Fat: 11.3 g, Protein: 44.3 g, Carbs: 6.9 g, Sodium: 541 mg

COOKING: 1H

PREPARATION: 15'

SERVES: 2

DIRECTIONS

1. Add all the ingredients to the slow cooker. Cook on low within 1 hour. Serve and enjoy.

DAY 6 — BREAKFAST

OATMEAL BANANA PANCAKES WITH WALNUTS

INGREDIENTS

- 1 finely diced firm banana
- 1 cup of whole wheat pancake mix
- 1/8 cup of chopped walnuts
- ¼ cup of old-fashioned oats

NUTRITIONAL FACTS:

Calories: 155, Fat: 4 g, Carbs: 28 g, Protein: 7 g, Sugars: 2.2 g, Sodium: 16 mg

COOKING: 5'

PREPARATION: 15'

SERVES: 8

DIRECTIONS

1. Make the pancake mix, as stated in the directions on the package. Add walnuts, oats, and chopped bananas. Coat a griddle with cooking spray. Add about ¼ cup of the pancake batter onto the grill when hot.
2. Turn pancake over when bubbles form on top. Cook until golden brown. Serve immediately.

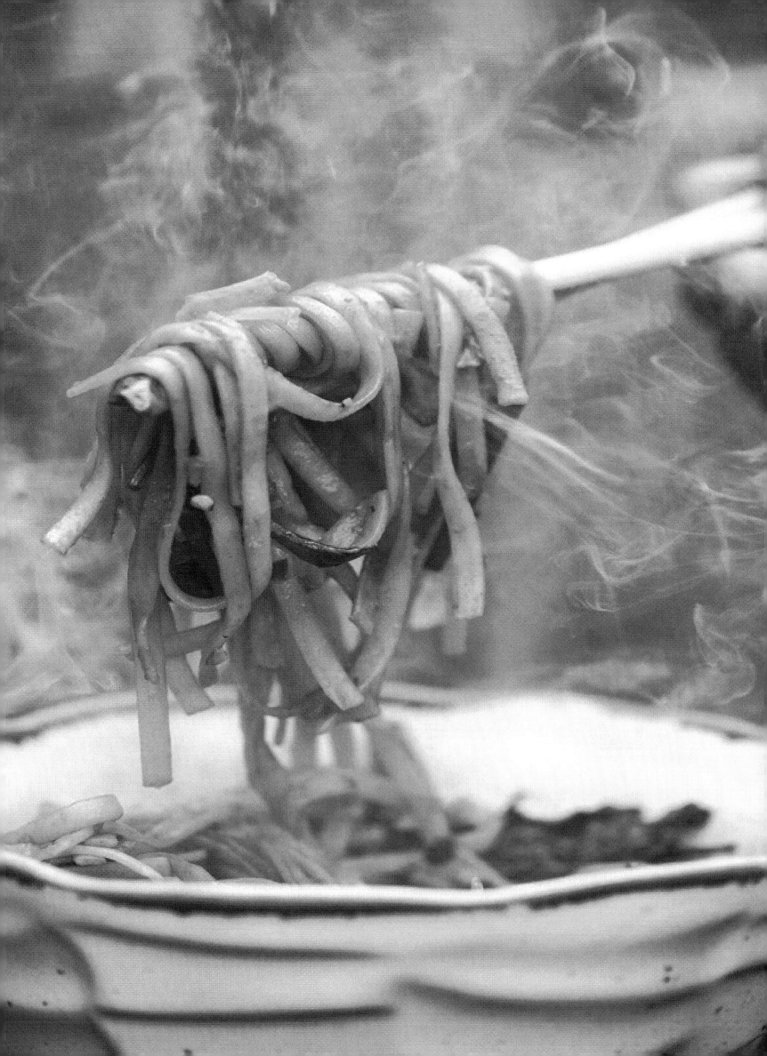

LUNCH

CURRY VEGETABLE NOODLES WITH CHICKEN

INGREDIENTS

- 21 ounces of zucchini
- 17 ounces of chicken fillet
- Pinch of salt and pepper
- 2 tablespoons of oil
- 5 ounces of red and yellow cherry tomatoes
- 1 teaspoon of curry powder
- 5 ounces of fat-free cheese
- 1 cup of vegetable broth
- 4 stalks of fresh basil

NUTRITIONAL FACTS:

Calories: 376, Fat: 17.2 g, Protein: 44.9 g, Sodium: 352 mg, Carbs: 9.5 g, Cholesterol: 53 mg

COOKING: 15'

PREPARATION: 15'

SERVES: 2

DIRECTIONS

1. Wash the zucchini, clean it, and cut it into long thin strips with a spiral cutter. Wash meat, pat dry, and season with salt. Heat 1 tbsp oil in a pan. Roast chicken in it for about 10 minutes until golden brown.

2. Wash cherry tomatoes and cut in half. Approximately 3 minutes before the end of the cooking time to the chicken in the pan. Heat 1 tablespoon of oil in another pan. Sweat curry powder into it, then stir in cream cheese and broth. Flavor the sauce with salt plus pepper and simmer for about 4 minutes.

3. Wash the basil, shake it dry and pluck the leaves from the stems. Cut small leaves of 3 stems. Remove meat from the pan and cut it into strips. Add tomatoes, basil, and zucchini to the sauce and heat for 2-3 minutes. Serve vegetable noodles and meat on plates and garnish with basil.

DINNER

OLIVE CAPERS CHICKEN

INGREDIENTS

- 2 lbs. of chicken
- 1/3 cup of chicken stock
- 3.5 ounces of Capers
- 6 ounces of olives
- ¼ cup of fresh basil
- 1 tablespoon of olive oil
- 1 teaspoon of oregano
- 2 garlic cloves, minced
- 2 tablespoons of red wine vinegar
- 1/8 teaspoon of pepper
- ¼ teaspoon of salt

NUTRITIONAL FACTS:

Calories: 433, Fat: 15.2 g, Protein: 66.9 g, Carbs: 4.8 g, Sodium 244 mg

COOKING: 16'

PREPARATION: 15'

SERVES: 4

DIRECTIONS

1. Put olive oil in your instant pot and set the pot on sauté mode. Add chicken to the pot and sauté for 3-4 minutes. Add remaining ingredients and stir well. Seal pot with the lid and select manual, and set timer for 12 minutes. Serve and enjoy.

DAY 7

BREAKFAST

SWEET BERRIES PANCAKE

INGREDIENTS

- 4 cups of almond flour
- Pinch of sea salt
- 2 organic eggs
- 4 teaspoons of walnut oil
- 1 cup of strawberries, mashed
- 1 cup of blueberries, mashed
- 1 teaspoon baking powder
- Honey for topping, optional

NUTRITIONAL FACTS:

Calories: 161, Carbs: 23 g, Fat: 6 g, Protein: 3 g, Cholesterol: 82 mg, Sodium: 91 mg, Potassium: 252 mg

COOKING: 15'

PREPARATION: 15'

SERVES: 4

DIRECTIONS

1. Take a bowl and add almond flour, baking powder, and sea salt. Take another bowl and add eggs, walnut oil, strawberries, and blueberries mash. Combine the ingredients of both bowls.

2. Heat a bit of walnut oil in a cooking pan and pour the spoonful mixture to make pancakes. Once the bubble comes on the top, flip the pancake to cook from the other side. Once done, serve with the glaze of honey on top.

LUNCH

BLACK BEAN STEW WITH CORNBREAD

INGREDIENTS

For the black bean stew:
- 2 tablespoons of canola oil
- 1 yellow onion, peeled and diced
- 4 garlic cloves, peeled and minced
- 1 tablespoon of chili powder
- 1 tablespoon of ground cumin
- ¼ teaspoon of kosher or sea salt
- ½ teaspoon of ground black pepper
- 2 cans of no-salt-added black beans, drained
- 1 (10-ounces) can fire-roasted diced tomatoes
- ½ cup of fresh cilantro leaves, chopped

For the cornbread topping:
- 1¼ cups of cornmeal
- ½ cup of all-purpose flour
- ½ teaspoon of baking powder
- ¼ teaspoon of baking soda
- 1/8 teaspoon of kosher or sea salt
- 1 cup of low-fat buttermilk
- 2 tablespoons of honey
- 1 large egg

NUTRITIONAL FACTS:

Calories: 359, Fat: 7 g, Sodium: 409 mg, Carbs: 61 g, Protein: 14 g

COOKING: 55'

PREPARATION: 15'

SERVES: 6

DIRECTIONS

1. Warm up the canola oil over medium heat in a large Dutch oven or stockpot. Add the onion and sauté for 4 to 6 minutes until the onion is soft. Stir in the garlic, chili powder, cumin, salt, and black pepper.

2. Cook within 1 to 2 minutes, until fragrant. Add the black beans and diced tomatoes. Bring to a simmer and cook for 15 minutes. Remove, then stir in the fresh cilantro. Taste and adjust the seasoning, if necessary.

3. Preheat the oven to 375 °F. While the stew simmers, prepare the cornbread topping. Mix the cornmeal, baking soda, flour, baking powder, plus salt in a bowl. In a measuring cup, whisk the buttermilk, honey, and egg until combined. Put the batter into the dry fixing until just combined.

4. In oven-safe bowls or dishes, spoon out the black bean soup. Distribute dollops of the cornbread batter on top and then spread it out evenly with a spatula. Bake within 30 minutes until the cornbread is just set.

DINNER

SOUTHWESTERN CHICKEN AND PASTA

INGREDIENTS

- 1 cup of uncooked whole-wheat rigatoni
- 2 chicken breasts, cut into cubes
- ¼ cup of salsa
- 1 ½ cups of canned unsalted tomato sauce
- 1/8 teaspoon of garlic powder
- 1 teaspoon of cumin
- ½ teaspoon of chili powder
- ½ cup of canned black beans, drained
- ½ cup of fresh corn
- ¼ cup of Monterey Jack and Colby cheese, shredded

NUTRITIONAL FACTS:

Calories: 245, Fat: 16.3 g, Sodium: 515 mg, Carbs: 19.3 g, Protein: 33.3 g

COOKING: 10'

PREPARATION: 10'

SERVES: 2

DIRECTIONS

1. Fill a pot with water up to ¾ full and boil it. Add pasta to cook until it is al dente, then drain the pasta while rinsing under cold water. Preheat a skillet with cooking oil, then cook the chicken for 10 minutes until golden from both sides.

2. Add tomato sauce, salsa, cumin, garlic powder, black beans, corn, and chili powder. Cook the mixture while stirring, then toss in the pasta. Serve with 2 tablespoons of cheese on top. Enjoy.

CHAPTER 6

MEAL PLAN WEEK 2

DAY 8

BREAKFAST

CARROT MUFFINS

INGREDIENTS

- 1 and ½ cups of whole wheat flour
- ½ cup of stevia
- 1 teaspoon of baking powder
- ½ teaspoon of cinnamon powder
- ½ teaspoon of baking soda
- ¼ cup of natural apple juice
- ¼ cup of olive oil
- 1 egg
- 1 cup of fresh cranberries
- 2 carrots, grated
- 2 teaspoons of ginger, grated
- ¼ cup of pecans, chopped
- Cooking spray

NUTRITIONAL FACTS:

Calories: 34, Carbs: 6 g, Fat: 1 g, Protein: 0 g, Sodium: 52 mg

COOKING: 30'

PREPARATION: 10'

SERVES: 5

DIRECTIONS

1. Mix the flour with the stevia, baking powder, cinnamon, and baking soda in a large bowl. Add the apple juice, oil, egg, cranberries, carrots, ginger, and pecans and stir well.

2. Oil a muffin tray with cooking spray, divide the muffin mix, put in the oven, and cook at 375 °F within 30 minutes. Divide the muffins between plates and serve for breakfast.

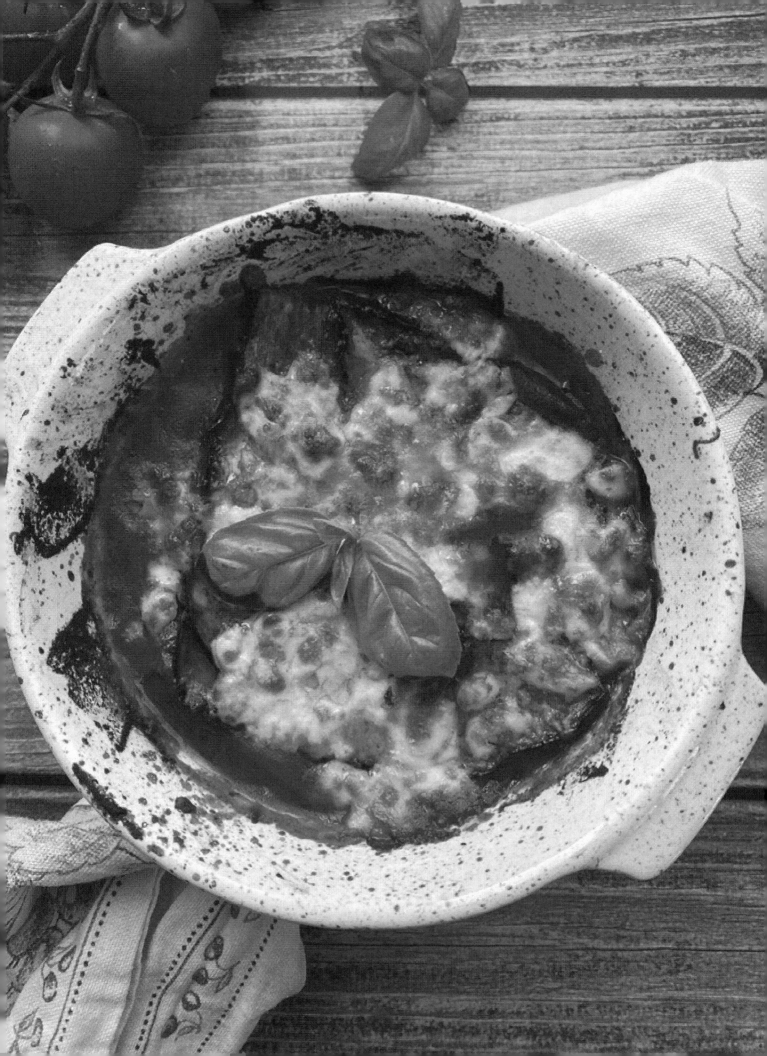

EGGPLANT PARMESAN STACKS

INGREDIENTS

- 1 large eggplant, cut into thick slices
- 2 tablespoons olive oil, divided
- ¼ teaspoon kosher or sea salt
- ¼ teaspoon ground black pepper
- 1 cup panko bread crumbs
- ¼ cup freshly grated Parmesan cheese
- 5 to 6 garlic cloves, minced
- ½ pound fresh mozzarella, sliced
- 1½ cups lower-sodium marinara
- ½ cup fresh basil leaves, torn

NUTRITIONAL FACTS:

Calories: 377, Fat: 22 g, Sodium: 509 mg, Carbs: 29 g, Protein: 16 g

COOKING: 20'

PREPARATION: 15'

SERVES: 4

DIRECTIONS

1. Preheat the oven to 425°F. Coat the eggplant slices in 1 tablespoon olive oil and sprinkle with salt and black pepper. Put on a large baking sheet, then roast for 10 to 12 minutes, until soft with crispy edges. Remove the eggplant and set the oven to low heat.

2. Stir the remaining tablespoon of olive oil, bread crumbs, Parmesan cheese, and garlic in a bowl. Remove the cooled eggplant from the baking sheet and clean it.

3. Create layers on the same baking sheet by stacking a roasted eggplant slice with a slice of mozzarella, a tablespoon of marinara, and a tablespoon of the bread crumb mixture, repeating with 2 layers of each ingredient. Cook under the broiler within 3 to 4 minutes until the cheese is melted and bubbly.

BEEF STEW WITH FENNEL AND SHALLOTS

INGREDIENTS

- 1 tablespoon of olive oil
- 1-pound of boneless lean beef stew meat, trimmed from fat and cut into cubes
- ½ fennel bulb, trimmed and sliced thinly
- 3 large shallots, chopped
- ¾ teaspoons of ground black pepper
- 2 fresh thyme sprigs
- 1 bay leaf
- 3 cups of low sodium beef broth
- ½ cup of red wine
- 4 large carrots, peeled and cut into chunks
- 4 large white potatoes, peeled and cut into chunks
- 3 portobello mushrooms, cleaned and cut into chunks
- 1/3 cup of Italian parsley, chopped

NUTRITIONAL FACTS:

Calories: 244, Protein: 21 g, Carbs: 22 g, Fat: 8 g, Saturated Fat: 2 g, Sodium: 184 mg

COOKING: 40'

PREPARATION: 10'

SERVES: 6

DIRECTIONS

1. Heat oil in a pot over medium heat and stir in the beef cubes for 5 minutes or until all sides turn brown.
2. Stir in the fennel, shallots, black pepper, and thyme for one minute or until the ingredients become fragrant.
3. Stir in the bay leaf, broth, red wine, carrots, white potatoes, and mushrooms.
4. Bring to a boil and cook for 30 minutes or until everything is tender.
5. Stir in the parsley last.

DAY 9

BREAKFAST

PUMPKIN MUFFINS

INGREDIENTS

- 4 cups of almond flour
- 2 cups of pumpkin, cooked and pureed
- 2 large whole organic eggs
- 3 teaspoons of baking powder
- 2 teaspoons of ground cinnamon
- ½ cup of raw honey
- 4 teaspoons of almond butter

NUTRITIONAL FACTS:

Calories: 136, Carbs: 22 g, Fat: 5 g, Protein: 2 g, Sodium: 11 mg, Potassium: 699 mg

COOKING: 20'

PREPARATION: 15'

SERVES: 4

DIRECTIONS

1. Preheat the oven at 400 °F. Line the muffin paper on the muffin tray. Mix the almond flour, pumpkin puree, eggs, baking powder, cinnamon, almond butter, and honey in a large bowl.
2. Put the prepared batter into a muffin tray and bake within 20 minutes. Once golden-brown, serve and enjoy.

LUNCH

DILL AND LEMON COD PACKETS

INGREDIENTS

- » 2 teaspoons of olive oil, divided
- » 4 slices of lemon, divided
- » 2 sprigs of fresh dill, divided
- » ½ teaspoon of garlic powder, divided
- » Pepper to taste
- » ½ lb. of cod filets

NUTRITIONAL FACTS:

Calories: 164,8 g, Carbs: 9.4 g, Protein: 18.3 g, Fats: 6 g, Sodium: 347 mg

COOKING: 10'

PREPARATION: 15'

SERVES: 2

DIRECTIONS

1. Cut 2 pieces of 15-inch lengths foil. Put one filet in the middle in one foil. Season with pepper to taste. Sprinkle ¼ teaspoon of garlic. Add a teaspoon of oil on top of the filet. Top with 2 slices of lemon and a sprig of dill.

2. Fold over the foil and seal the filet inside. Repeat the process for the rest of the fish. Place packet on the trivet. Cover and steam for 10 minutes. Serve.

DINNER   DASH DIET 2022

STUFFED CHICKEN BREASTS

INGREDIENTS

- 3 tablespoons of seedless raisins
- ½ cup of chopped onion
- ½ cup of chopped celery
- ¼ teaspoon of garlic, minced
- 1 bay leaf
- 1 cup of apple with peel, chopped
- 2 tablespoons of chopped water chestnuts
- 4 large chicken breast halves, 5 Ounces of each
- 1 tablespoon of olive oil
- 1 cup of fat-free milk
- 1 teaspoon of curry powder
- 2 tablespoons of all-purpose (plain) flour
- 1 lemon, cut into 4 wedges

NUTRITIONAL FACTS:

Calories: 357, Fat: 32.7 g, Sodium: 277 mg, Carbs: 17.7 g, Protein: 31.2 g

COOKING: 30'

PREPARATION: 15'

SERVES: 4

DIRECTIONS

1. Set the oven to heat at 425 °F. Grease a baking dish with cooking oil. Soak raisins in warm water until they swell. Grease a heated skillet with cooking spray.

2. Add the celery, garlic, onions, and bay leaf. Sauté for 5 minutes. Discard the bay leaf, then toss in apples. Stir cook for 2 minutes. Drain the soaked raisin and pat them dry to remove excess water.

3. Add raisins and water chestnuts to the apple mixture. Pull apart the chicken's skin and stuff the apple raisin mixture between the skin and the chicken. Preheat olive oil in another skillet and sear the breasts for 5 minutes per side.

4. Place the chicken breasts in the baking dish and cover the dish. Bake for 15 minutes until temperature reaches 165 °F. Prepare sauce by mixing milk, flour, and curry powder in a saucepan.

5. Stir cook until the mixture thickens, about 5 minutes. Pour this sauce over the baked chicken. Bake again in the covered dish for 10 minutes. Serve.

DASH DIET 2022

DAY 10

BREAKFAST

APPLE PANCAKES

INGREDIENTS

- ¼ cup of extra-virgin olive oil, divided
- 1 cup of whole wheat flour
- 2 teaspoons of baking powder
- 1 teaspoon of baking soda
- 1 teaspoon of ground cinnamon
- 1 cup of 1% milk
- 2 large eggs
- 1 medium Gala apple, diced
- 2 tablespoons of maple syrup
- ¼ cup of chopped walnuts

NUTRITIONAL FACTS:

Calories: 378, Carbs: 39 g, Fat: 22 g, Protein: 10 g, Sodium: 65 mg

COOKING: **5'**

PREPARATION: **15'**

SERVES: **16**

DIRECTIONS

1. Set aside 1 teaspoon of oil to use for greasing a griddle or skillet. Stir the flour, baking powder, baking soda, cinnamon, milk, eggs, apple, and the remaining oil in a large bowl.

2. Warm the griddle or skillet on medium-high heat and coat with the reserved oil. Working in batches, pour in about ¼ cup of the batter for each pancake. Cook until browned on both sides.

3. Place 4 pancakes into each of 4 medium storage containers and the maple syrup in 4 small containers. Put each serving with 1 tablespoon of walnuts and drizzle with ½ tablespoon of maple syrup.

LUNCH

SALMON WRAP

INGREDIENTS

- 2 ounces of Smoked Salmon
- 2 teaspoons of low-fat cream cheese
- ½ medium-size red onion, finely sliced
- ½ teaspoon of fresh basil or dried basil
- Pinch of pepper
- Arugula leaves
- 1 Homemade wrap or any whole-meal tortilla

NUTRITIONAL FACTS:

Calories: 151, Carbs: 19.2 g, Fat: 3.4 g, Protein: 10.4 g, Sodium: 316 mg

COOKING: 0'

PREPARATION: 15'

SERVES: 1

DIRECTIONS

1. Warm the wraps or tortillas into a heated pan or oven. Combine the cream cheese, basil, pepper, and spread into the tortilla. Top with salmon, arugula, and sliced onion. Roll up and slice. Serve and Enjoy!

DINNER

HONEY CRUSTED CHICKEN

INGREDIENTS

- 1 teaspoon of paprika
- 8 saltine crackers, 2 inches square
- 2 chicken breasts, each 4 Ounces
- 4 teaspoons of honey

NUTRITIONAL FACTS:

Calories: 219, Fat: 17 g, Sodium: 456 mg, Carbs: 12.1 g, Protein: 31 g

COOKING: 25'

PREPARATION: 10'

SERVES: 2

DIRECTIONS

1. Set the oven to heat at 375 °F. Grease a baking dish with cooking oil. Smash the crackers in a Ziploc bag and toss them with paprika in a bowl. Brush chicken with honey and add it to the crackers.

2. Mix well and transfer the chicken to the baking dish. Bake the chicken for 25 minutes until golden brown. Serve.

DAY 11 — BREAKFAST

STRAWBERRY SANDWICH

INGREDIENTS

- 8 ounces of low-fat cream cheese, soft
- 1 Tablespoon of stevia
- 1 teaspoon of lemon zest, grated
- 4 whole-wheat English muffins, toasted
- 2 cups of strawberries, sliced

NUTRITIONAL FACTS:

Calories: 150, Carbs: 23 g, Fat: 7 g, Protein: 2 g, Sodium: 70 mg

COOKING: 0'

PREPARATION: 10'

SERVES: 4

DIRECTIONS

1. In your food processor, combine the cream cheese with the stevia and lemon zest and pulse well. Spread 1 tablespoon of this mix on 1 muffin half and top with some of the sliced strawberries. Repeat with the rest of the muffin halves and serve for breakfast. Enjoy!

LUNCH

SWEET POTATOES AND ZUCCHINI SOUP

INGREDIENTS

- 4 cups of veggie stock
- 2 tablespoons of olive oil
- 2 sweet potatoes, peeled and cubed
- 8 zucchinis, chopped
- 2 yellow onions, chopped
- 1 cup of coconut milk
- A pinch of black pepper
- 1 tablespoon of coconut aminos
- 4 tablespoons of dill, chopped
- ½ teaspoon of basil, chopped

NUTRITIONAL FACTS:

Calories: 270, Carbs: 50 g, Fat: 4 g, Protein: 11 g, Sodium: 416 mg

COOKING: **20'**

PREPARATION: **10'**

SERVES: **8**

DIRECTIONS

1. Heat a pot with the oil over medium heat, add onion, stir and cook for 5 minutes. Add zucchinis, stock, basil, potato, and pepper, stir and cook for 15 minutes more. Add milk, aminos, and dill, pulse using an immersion blender, ladle into bowls and serve for lunch.

DINNER

PORK AND ROASTED TOMATOES MIX

INGREDIENTS

- ½ cup of chopped yellow onion
- 2 cups of chopped zucchinis
- 1 lb. of ground pork meat
- ¾ cup of shredded low-fat cheddar cheese
- Black pepper
- 15 ounces of no-salt-added, chopped and canned roasted tomatoes

NUTRITIONAL FACTS:

Calories: 270, Fat: 5 g, Sodium: 390 mg, Carbs: 10 g, Sugars: 8 g, Protein: 12 g

COOKING: 15'

PREPARATION: 10'

SERVES: 6

DIRECTIONS

1. Heat a pan over medium-high heat, add the pork, onion, black pepper, and zucchini, stir and cook for 7 minutes.
2. Add the roasted tomatoes, stir, bring to a boil, cook over medium heat for 8 minutes, divide into bowls, sprinkle cheddar on the top, and serve.
3. Enjoy!

DASH DIET 2022

DAY 12

BREAKFAST

SCRAMBLED EGG AND VEGGIE BREAKFAST QUESADILLAS

INGREDIENTS

- 2 eggs
- 2 egg whites
- 2 to 4 tablespoons of nonfat or low-fat milk
- ¼ teaspoon of freshly ground black pepper
- 1 large tomato, chopped
- 2 tablespoons of chopped cilantro
- ½ cup of canned black beans, rinsed and drained
- 1½ tablespoons of olive oil, divided
- 4 corn tortillas
- ½ avocado, peeled, pitted, and thinly sliced

NUTRITIONAL FACTS:

Calories: 445, Carbs: 42 g, Fat: 24 g, Fiber: 11 g, Protein: 19 g, Sodium: 228 mg, Potassium: 614 mg, Sugars: 2 g

COOKING: 15'

PREPARATION: 15'

SERVES: 2

DIRECTIONS

1. Mix the eggs, egg whites, milk, and black pepper in a bowl. Using an electric mixer, beat until smooth. Add the tomato, cilantro, and black beans to the same bowl, and fold into the eggs with a spoon.

2. Warm half of the olive oil in a medium pan over medium heat. Add the scrambled egg mixture and cook for a few minutes, stirring, until cooked through. Remove from the pan.

3. Divide the scrambled-egg mixture between the tortillas, layering only on one half of the tortilla. Top with avocado slices and fold the tortillas in half.

4. Heat the remaining oil over medium heat, and add one of the folded tortillas to the pan. Cook within 1 to 2 minutes on each side or until browned. Repeat with remaining tortillas. Serve immediately.

LUNCH

CHICKPEA CAULIFLOWER TIKKA MASALA

INGREDIENTS

- 2 tablespoons of olive oil
- 1 yellow onion, peeled and diced
- 4 garlic cloves, peeled and minced
- 1-inch piece of fresh ginger, peeled and minced
- 2 tablespoons of Garam Masala
- 1 teaspoon of kosher or sea salt
- ½ Teaspoon of ground black pepper
- ¼ teaspoon of ground cayenne pepper
- ½ small head cauliflower, small florets
- 2 (15 ounces) cans of no-salt-added chickpeas, rinsed and drained
- 1 (15 ounces) can no-salt-added petite diced tomatoes, drained
- 1½ cups of unsalted vegetable broth
- ½ (15 ounces) can coconut milk
- Zest and juice of 1 lime
- ½ cup of fresh cilantro leaves, chopped, divided
- 1½ cup of cooked Fluffy Brown Rice, divided

NUTRITIONAL FACTS:

Calories: 323, Fat: 12 g, Sodium: 444 mg, Carbs: 44 g, Protein: 11 g

COOKING: 40'

PREPARATION: 15'

SERVES: 6

DIRECTIONS

1. Warm the olive oil over medium heat, then put the onion and sauté within 4 to 5 minutes in a large Dutch oven or stockpot. Stir in the garlic, ginger, garam masala, salt, black pepper, and cayenne pepper and toast for 30 to 60 seconds, until fragrant.

2. Stir in the cauliflower florets, chickpeas, diced tomatoes, and vegetable broth and increase to medium-high. Simmer within 15 minutes until the cauliflower is fork-tender.

3. Remove, then stir in the coconut milk, lime juice, lime zest, and half of the cilantro. Taste and adjust the seasoning, if necessary. Serve over the rice and the remaining chopped cilantro.

DINNER

EASY SHRIMP

INGREDIENTS

- 1-pound of cooked shrimp
- 1 pack of mixed frozen vegetables
- 1 garlic clove, minced
- 1 teaspoon of butter or margarine
- ¼ cup of water
- 1 package of shrimp-flavored instant noodles
- 3 teaspoons of low sodium soy sauce
- ½ teaspoon of ground ginger
- Salt and pepper, to taste

NUTRITIONAL FACTS:

Calories: 80, Protein: 18.9 g, Carbs: 62 g, Fat: 9 g, Sodium: 276 mg

COOKING: 10'

PREPARATION: 15'

SERVES: 4

DIRECTIONS

1. In a large skillet, melt the butter. Add the minced garlic, sweat it for 1 minute. Add the shrimp and vegetables to the skillet. Add soy sauce and ginger. Season with salt and pepper. Cover and simmer for 5 - 10 minutes, until the shrimp turns pink and the vegetables are tender.

2. Boil water in a separate pot. Add the noodles. Turn off the heat, cover the pot. Let it stand for 3 minutes. (Keep the water.)

3. Using a scoop or tongs, transfer the noodles to the skillet with the shrimp and vegetables. Stir in the seasoning packet. Mix, then serve immediately.

DAY 13

DASH DIET 2022

BREAKFAST

ENERGY SUNRISE MUFFINS

INGREDIENTS

- Nonstick cooking spray
- 2 cups of whole wheat flour
- 2 teaspoons of baking soda
- 2 teaspoons of ground cinnamon
- 1 teaspoon of ground ginger
- ¼ teaspoon of salt
- 3 large eggs
- ½ cup of packed brown sugar
- 1/3 cup of unsweetened applesauce
- ¼ cup of honey
- ¼ cup of vegetable or canola oil
- 1 teaspoon of grated orange zest
- Juice of 1 medium orange
- 2 teaspoons of vanilla extract
- 2 cups of shredded carrots
- 1 large apple, peeled and grated
- ½ cup of golden raisins
- ½ cup of chopped pecans
- ½ cup of unsweetened coconut flakes

NUTRITIONAL FACTS:

Calories: 292, Fat: 14 g, Carbs: 42 g, Protein: 5 g, Sodium: 84 mg

COOKING: 25'

PREPARATION: 15'

SERVES: 16

DIRECTIONS

1. If you can fit two 12-cup muffin tins side by side in your oven, then leave a rack in the middle, then preheat the oven to 350 °F.

2. Coat 16 cups of the muffin tins with cooking spray or line with paper liners. Mix the flour, baking soda, cinnamon, ginger, and salt in a large bowl. Set aside.

3. Mix the eggs, brown sugar, applesauce, honey, oil, orange zest, orange juice, and vanilla until combined in a medium bowl. Add the carrots and apple and whisk again.

4. Mix the dry and wet ingredients with a spatula. Fold in the raisins, pecans, and coconut. Mix everything once again, just until well combined. Put the batter into the prepared muffin cups, filling them to the top.

5. Bake within 20 to 25 minutes, or until a wooden toothpick inserted into the middle of the center muffin comes out clean (switching racks halfway through if baking on 2 racks). Cool for 5 minutes in the tins, then transfer to a wire rack to cool for an additional 5 minutes. Cool completely before storing in containers.

MEXICAN-STYLE POTATO CASSEROLE

INGREDIENTS

- Cooking spray
- 2 tablespoons of canola oil
- ½ yellow onion, peeled and diced
- 4 garlic cloves, peeled and minced
- 2 tablespoons of all-purpose flour
- 1¼ cups of milk
- 1 tablespoon of chili powder
- ½ Tablespoon of ground cumin
- 1 teaspoon of kosher salt or sea salt
- ½ teaspoon of ground black pepper
- ¼ teaspoon of ground cayenne pepper
- 1½ cups of shredded Mexican-style cheese, divided
- 1 (4 ounces) can green chilis, drained
- 1 ½ pound of baby Yukon Gold or red potatoes, thinly sliced
- 1 red bell pepper, thinly sliced

NUTRITIONAL FACTS:

Calories: 195, Fat: 10 g, Sodium: 487 mg, Carbs: 19 g, Protein: 8 g

COOKING: 60'

PREPARATION: 15'

SERVES: 8

DIRECTIONS

1. Preheat the oven to 400 °F. Oiled a 9-by-13-inch baking dish with cooking spray. In a large saucepan, warm canola oil on medium heat. Add the onion and sauté for 4 to 5 minutes, until soft. Mix in the garlic, then cook until fragrant, 30 to 60 seconds.

2. Mix in the flour, then put in the milk while whisking. Slow simmer for about 5 minutes until thickened. Whisk in the chili powder, cumin, salt, black pepper, and cayenne pepper.

3. Remove from the heat and whisk in half of the shredded cheese and the green chilis. Taste and adjust the seasoning, if necessary. Line up one-third of the sliced potatoes and sliced bell pepper in the baking dish and top with a quarter of the remaining shredded cheese.

4. Repeat with 2 more layers. Pour the cheese sauce over the top and sprinkle with the remaining shredded cheese. Cover it with aluminum foil and bake within 45 to 50 minutes until the potatoes are tender.

5. Remove the foil and bake again within 5 to 10 minutes, until the topping is slightly browned. Let cool within 20 minutes before slicing into 8 pieces. Serve.

DINNER

BASIL HALIBUT

INGREDIENTS

- 4 Halibut Fillets, 4 ounces of each
- 2 teaspoons of olive oil
- 1 tablespoon of garlic, minced
- 2 tomatoes, diced
- 2 tablespoons of basil, fresh & chopped
- 1 teaspoon of oregano, fresh & chopped

NUTRITIONAL FACTS:

Calories: 128, Protein: 21 g, Fat: 4 g, Carbs: 3 g, Sodium: 81 mg, Cholesterol: 55 mg

COOKING: 20'

PREPARATION: 10'

SERVES: 4

DIRECTIONS

1. Heat the oven to 350 °F, and then get out a 9 by 13-inch pan. Spray it down with cooking spray.
2. Toss the basil, olive oil, garlic, oregano, and tomato together in a bowl. Pour this over your fish in the pan.
3. Bake for 12 minutes. Your fish should be flakey.

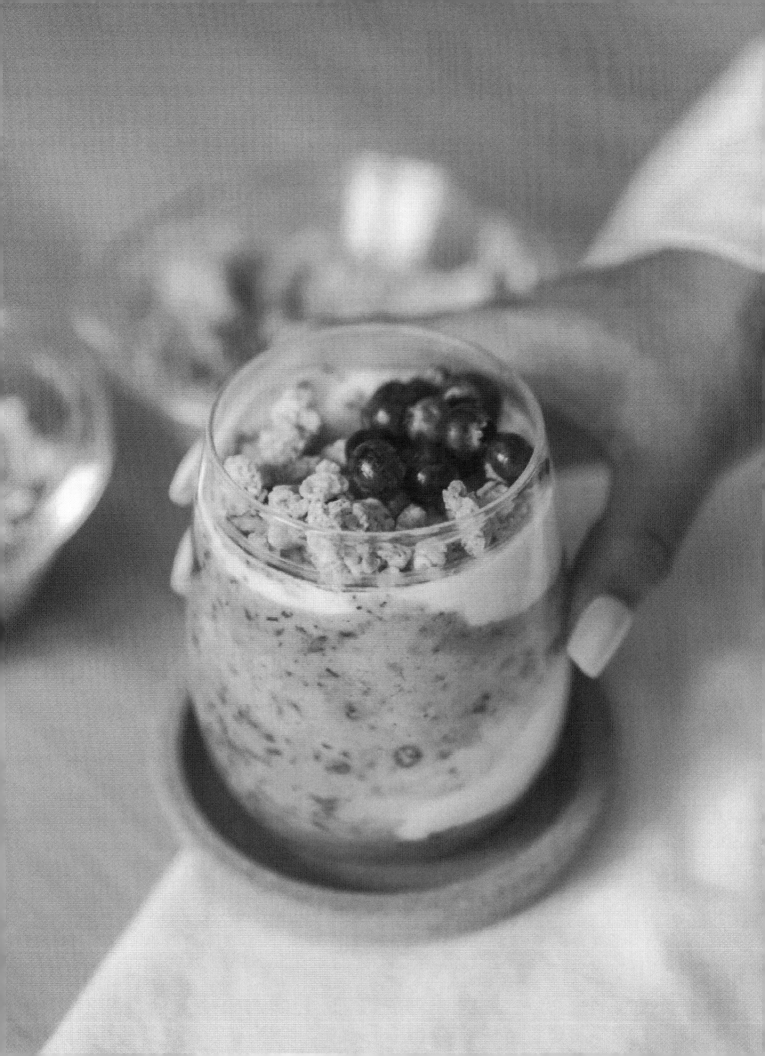

DAY 14 — DASH DIET 2022

BREAKFAST

CREAMY OATS & BLUEBERRY SMOOTHIE

INGREDIENTS

- 1 cup of cold Fat-free milk
- ½ cup of fresh frozen blueberries
- ½ cup of frozen cooked oatmeal
- 1 tablespoon of sunflower seeds

NUTRITIONAL FACTS:

Calories: 280, Fat: 6.8 g, Carbs: 44.0 g, Protein: 14.0 g, Sugars: 32 g, Sodium: 141 mg

COOKING: 0'

PREPARATION: 4'

SERVES: 1

DIRECTIONS

1. Blend all the ingredients using a powerful blender until smooth and creamy. Serve and enjoy.

LUNCH

DILL CHICKEN SALAD

INGREDIENTS

- 1 tablespoon of unsalted butter
- 1 small onion, diced
- 2 cloves of garlic, minced
- 500 g of boneless skinless chicken breasts

Salad:

- 2/3 cup of Fat-free yogurt
- ¼ cup of mayonnaise light
- 2 large shallots, minced
- ½ cup of fresh dill, finely chopped

NUTRITIONAL FACTS:

Calories: 253, Carbs: 9 g, Protein: 33.1 g, Fat: 9.5 g, Sodium: 236 mg

COOKING: 15'

PREPARATION: 15'

SERVES: 3

DIRECTIONS

1. Dissolve the butter over medium heat in a wide pan. Sauté the onion and garlic in the butter and chicken breasts. Put water to cover the chicken breasts by 1 inch. Bring to boil. Cover and reduce the heat to a bare simmer.

2. Cook within 8 to 10 minutes or until the chicken is cooked through. Cool thoroughly. The shred chicken finely using 2 forks. Set aside. Whisk the yogurt and mayonnaise. Then toss with the chicken. Add shallots and dill. Mix again all. Serve and Enjoy!

DINNER

WHITE BEANS WITH SPINACH AND PAN-ROASTED TOMATOES QUESADILLASVEGETABLE

INGREDIENTS

- 1 tablespoon of olive oil
- 4 small plum tomatoes, halved lengthwise
- 10 ounces of frozen spinach, defrosted and squeezed of excess water
- 2 garlic cloves, thinly sliced
- 2 tablespoons of water
- ¼ teaspoon of freshly ground black pepper
- 1 can of white beans, drained
- Juice of 1 lemon

NUTRITIONAL FACTS:

Calories: 293, Fat: 9 g, Sodium: 267 mg, Carbs: 43 g, Protein: 15 g

COOKING: 10'

PREPARATION: 15'

SERVES: 2

DIRECTIONS

1. Heat the oil in a large skillet over medium-high heat. Put the tomatoes, cut-side down, and cook within 3 to 5 minutes; turn and cook within 1 minute more. Transfer to a plate.

2. Reduce heat to medium and add the spinach, garlic, water, and pepper to the skillet. Cook, tossing until the spinach is heated through, 2 to 3 minutes.

3. Return the tomatoes to the skillet, put the white beans and lemon juice, and toss until heated through 1 to 2 minutes.

CHAPTER 7

MEAL PLAN WEEK 3

DAY 15

BREAKFAST

SPINACH, EGG, AND CHEESE BREAKFAST QUESADILLAS VEGETABLE

INGREDIENTS

- 1½ tablespoon of extra-virgin olive oil
- ½ medium onion, diced
- 1 medium red bell pepper, diced
- 4 large eggs
- 1/8 teaspoon of salt
- 1/8 teaspoon of freshly ground black pepper
- 4 cups of baby spinach
- ½ cup of crumbled feta cheese
- Nonstick cooking spray
- 4 (6-inches) of whole-wheat tortillas, divided
- 1 cup of shredded part-skim low-moisture mozzarella cheese, divided

NUTRITIONAL FACTS:

Calories: 453, Fat: 28 g, Carbs: 28 g, Fiber: 4.5 g, Protein: 23 g, Potassium: 205 mg, Sodium: 837 mg

COOKING: 15'

PREPARATION: 15'

SERVES: 4

DIRECTIONS

1. If you can fit two 12-cup muffin tins side by side in your oven, then leave a rack in the middle, then preheat the oven to 350 °F.

2. Coat 16 cups of the muffin tins with cooking spray or line with paper liners. Mix the flour, baking soda, cinnamon, ginger, and salt in a large bowl. Set aside.

3. Mix the eggs, brown sugar, applesauce, honey, oil, orange zest, orange juice, and vanilla until combined in a medium bowl. Add the carrots and apple and whisk again.

4. Mix the dry and wet ingredients with a spatula. Fold in the raisins, pecans, and coconut. Mix everything once again, just until well combined. Put the batter into the prepared muffin cups, filling them to the top.

5. Bake within 20 to 25 minutes, or until a wooden toothpick inserted into the middle of the center muffin comes out clean (switching racks halfway through if baking on 2 racks). Cool for 5 minutes in the tins, then transfer to a wire rack to cool for an additional 5 minutes. Cool completely before storing in containers.

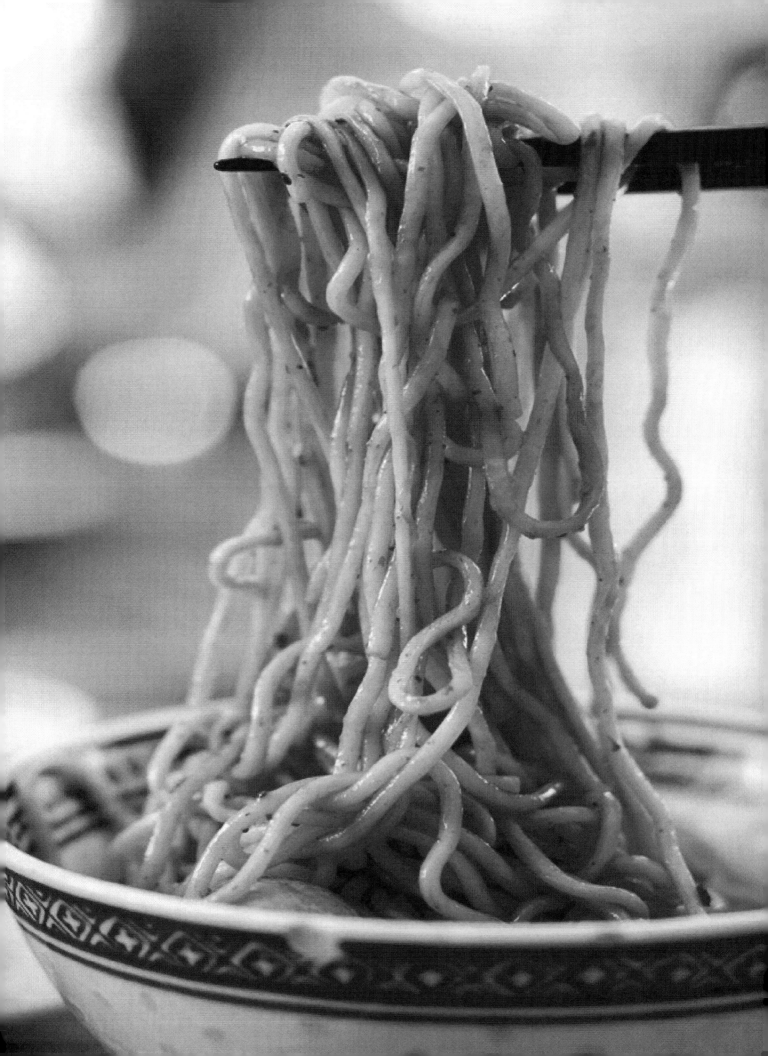

SWEET AND SOUR CHICKEN WHIT NOODLES AND VEGETABLE

INGREDIENTS

- 4 chicken fillets (75 g each)
- 300 g of whole-wheat spaghetti
- 750 g carrots
- ½ liter of clear chicken broth (instant)
- 1 tablespoon of sugar
- 1 tablespoon of green peppercorns
- 2-3 tablespoons of balsamic vinegar
- Pinch of salt

NUTRITIONAL FACTS:

Calories: 374, Fat: 21 g, Protein: 44 g, Sodium: 295 mg, Carbs: 23.1 g

COOKING: 30'

PREPARATION: 15'

SERVES: 4

DIRECTIONS

1. Cook the spaghetti in boiling water for about 8 minutes. Then drain. In the meantime, peel and wash carrots. Cut into long strips (best with a special grater). Blanch within 2 minutes in boiling salted water, drain. Wash the chicken fillets. Add to the boiling chicken soup and cook for about 15 minutes.

2. Melt the sugar until golden brown. Measure ¼ liter of chicken stock and deglaze the sugar with it. Add peppercorns, cook for 2 minutes. Season with salt and vinegar. Add the fillets, then cut into thin slices. Then turn the pasta and carrots in the sauce and serve garnished with capuchin blossoms. Serve and enjoy.

DINNER

LEEK & CAULIFLOWER SOUP

INGREDIENTS

- 1 tablespoon of olive oil
- 1 leek, trimmed & sliced thin
- 1 yellow onion, peeled & diced
- 1 head of cauliflower, chopped into florets
- 3 cloves of garlic, minced
- 2 tablespoons of thyme, fresh & chopped
- 1 teaspoon of Smoked Paprika
- 1 ¼ teaspoon of Sea Salt, Fine
- ¼ teaspoon of ground cayenne pepper
- 1 tablespoon of heavy cream
- 3 cups of vegetable stock, unsalted
- ½ lemon, juiced & zested

NUTRITIONAL FACTS:

Calories: 92, Protein: 5 g, Fat: 4 g, Carbs: 13 g, Sodium: 556 mg, Cholesterol: 3 mg

COOKING: 20'

PREPARATION: 20'

SERVES: 6

DIRECTIONS

1. Heat your oil in a stockpot over medium heat, and add in your leek, onion, and cauliflower. Cook for 5 minutes or until the onion begins to soften. Add your garlic, thyme, smoked paprika, salt, pepper, and cayenne. Pour in your vegetable stock and bring it to a simmer, cooking for 15 minutes. Your cauliflower should be very tender.

2. Remove from heat and stir in your lemon juice, lemon zest, and cream. Use an immersion blender to puree and serve warm.

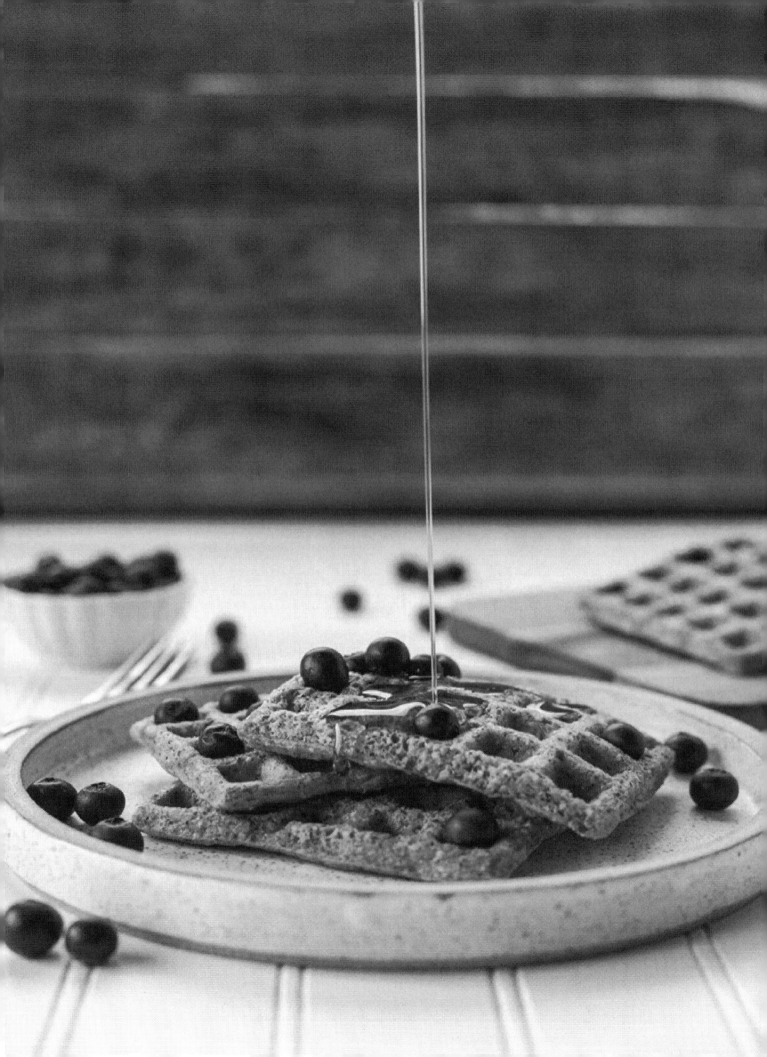

DAY 16

BREAKFAST

BLUEBERRY WAFFLES

INGREDIENTS

- 2 cups of whole wheat flour
- 1 tablespoon of baking powder
- 1 teaspoon of ground cinnamon
- 2 tablespoons of sugar
- 2 large eggs
- 3 tablespoons of unsalted butter, melted
- 3 tablespoons of nonfat plain Greek yogurt
- 1½ cups of 1% milk
- 2 teaspoons of vanilla extract
- 4 ounces of blueberries
- Nonstick cooking spray
- ½ cup of maple almond butter

NUTRITIONAL FACTS:

Calories: 647, Fat: 37 g, Carbs: 67 g, Protein: 22 g, Sodium: 156 mg

COOKING: 15'

PREPARATION: 15'

SERVES: 8

DIRECTIONS

1. Preheat the waffle iron. Mix the flour, baking powder, cinnamon, plus sugar in a large bowl. Mix the eggs, melted butter, yogurt, milk, and vanilla in a small bowl. Combine well.

2. Put the wet fixing to the dry mix and whisk until well combined. Do not over whisk; it's okay if the mixture has some lumps. Fold in the blueberries.

3. Oiled the waffle iron with cooking spray, then cook 1/3 cup of the batter until the waffles are lightly browned and slightly crisp. Repeat with the rest of the batter.

4. Place 2 waffles in each of 4 storage containers. Store the almond butter in 4 condiment cups. To serve, top each warm waffle with 1 tablespoon of maple almond butter.

LUNCH

STEAMED SALMON TERIYAKI

INGREDIENTS

- 3 green onions, minced
- 2 packets of Stevia
- 1 tablespoon of freshly grated ginger
- 1 clove of garlic, minced
- 2 teaspoons of sesame seeds
- 1 tablespoon of sesame oil
- ¼ cup of mirin
- 2 tablespoons of low sodium soy sauce
- ½ lb of salmon filet

NUTRITIONAL FACTS:

Calories: 242.7, Fat: 10.7 g, Sodium: 285 mg, Carbs: 1.2 g, Protein: 35.4 g

COOKING: 15'

PREPARATION: 15'

SERVES: 4

DIRECTIONS

1. Mix the stevia, ginger, garlic, oil, mirin, and soy sauce in a heat-proof dish that fits inside a saucepan. Add the salmon and cover generously with sauce.

2. Put the sesame seeds and green onions on top of the salmon. Cover the dish with foil. Place on top of the trivet. Cover and steam for 15 minutes. Let it rest for 5 minutes in the pan. Serve and enjoy.

DINNER

PORK MEDALLIONS WITH FIVE SPICE POWDER

INGREDIENTS

- 1 tablespoon of olive oil
- 3 cloves of garlic, minced
- 1-pound of pork tenderloin, fat trimmed
- 2 tablespoons of low-sodium soy sauce
- 1 tablespoon of green onion, minced
- ¾ teaspoon of five-spice powder
- ½ cup of water
- ¼ cup of dry white wine
- 1/3 cup of chopped onion
- ½ head green cabbage, thinly sliced and wilted
- 1 tablespoon of chopped fresh parsley

NUTRITIONAL FACTS:

Calories: 219, Protein: 25 g, Carbs: 5 g, Fat: 11 g, Saturated Fat: 2 g, Sodium: 296 mg

COOKING: 25'

PREPARATION: 10'

SERVES: 4

DIRECTIONS

1. Combine the olive oil, garlic, pork tenderloin, soy sauce, green onion, and five-spice powder in a bowl. Mix until well combined and allow to marinate in the fridge for at least 2 hours.

2. Heat the oven to 400 °F.

3. Remove the pork from the marinade and pat dry.

4. On a skillet, sear the meat on all sides until slightly brown before transferring it into a heat-proof baking dish.

5. Place inside the oven and roast the pork for 20 minutes.

6. Meanwhile, pour the water, dry white wine, and onions in the skillet where you seared the pork and deglaze. Allow simmering until the sauce has reduced.

7. Serve the pork medallions with wilted cabbages and parsley and drizzle the sauce on top.

DASH DIET 2022

DAY 17

BREAKFAST

SUPER-SIMPLE GRANOLA

INGREDIENTS

- ¼ cup of extra-virgin olive oil
- ¼ cup of honey
- ½ teaspoon of ground cinnamon
- ½ teaspoon of vanilla extract
- ¼ teaspoon of salt
- 2 cups of rolled oats
- ½ cup of chopped walnuts
- ½ cup of slivered almonds

NUTRITIONAL FACTS:

Calories: 254, Fat: 16 g, Carbs: 25 g, Fiber: 3.5 g, Protein: 5 g, Potassium: 163 mg, Sodium: 73 mg

COOKING: 25'

PREPARATION: 15'

SERVES: 8

DIRECTIONS

1. Preheat the oven to 350 °F. Mix the oil, honey, cinnamon, vanilla, and salt in a large bowl. Add the oats, walnuts, and almonds. Stir to coat. Put the batter out onto the prepared sheet pan. Bake for 20 minutes. Let cool.

LUNCH

LIGHT BALSAMIC SALAD

INGREDIENTS

- 1 orange, cut into segments
- 2 green onions, chopped
- 1 romaine lettuce head, torn
- 1 avocado, pitted, peeled, and cubed
- ¼ cup of almonds, sliced

For the salad dressing:

- 1 teaspoon of mustard
- ¼ cup of olive oil
- 2 tablespoons of balsamic vinegar
- ½ Juice of orange
- Salt and black pepper

NUTRITIONAL FACTS:

Calories: 35, Carbs: 5 g, Fat: 2 g, Protein: 0 g, Sodium 400 mg

COOKING: 0'

PREPARATION: 10'

SERVES: 3

DIRECTIONS

1. In a salad bowl, mix oranges with avocado, lettuce, almonds, and green onions. In another bowl, mix olive oil with vinegar, mustard, orange juice, salt, and pepper, whisk well, add this to your salad, toss and serve.

DINNER

MUSTARD CHICKEN TENDERS

INGREDIENTS

- 1 lb. of chicken tenders
- 2 tablespoons of fresh tarragon, chopped
- ½ cup of whole-grain mustard
- ½ teaspoon of paprika
- 1 garlic clove, minced
- ½ ounce of fresh lemon juice
- ½ teaspoon of pepper
- ¼ teaspoon of kosher salt

NUTRITIONAL FACTS:

Calories: 242, Fat: 9.5 g, Protein: 33.2 g, Carbs: 3.1 g, Sodium: 240 mg

COOKING: 20'

PREPARATION: 15'

SERVES: 4

DIRECTIONS

1. Warm the oven to 425 °F. Add all the ingredients except chicken to the large bowl and mix well. Put the chicken in the bowl, then stir until well coated. Place chicken on a baking dish and cover. Bake within 15-20 minutes. Serve and enjoy.

DAY 18

DASH DIET 2022

BREAKFAST

BREAKFAST BANANA SPLIT

INGREDIENTS

- 2 bananas, peeled
- 1 cup of oats, cooked
- ½ cup of low-fat strawberry yogurt
- 1/3 teaspoon of honey, optional
- ½ cup of pineapple, chunks

NUTRITIONAL FACTS:

Calories: 145, Protein: 3 g, Carbs: 18 g, Fat: 7 g, Sodium: 2 mg, Potassium: 380 mg

COOKING: 0'

PREPARATION: 15'

SERVES: 3

DIRECTIONS

1. Peel the bananas and cut lengthwise. Place half of the banana in each separate bowl. Spoon strawberry yogurt on top and pour cooked oats with pineapple chunks on each banana. Serve immediately with a glaze of honey of liked.

LUNCH

LEMONGRASS AND CHICKEN SOUP

INGREDIENTS

- 4 lime leaves, torn
- 4 cups of veggie stock, low-sodium
- 1 lemongrass stalk, chopped
- 1 tablespoon of ginger, grated
- 1 pound of chicken breast, skinless, boneless, and cubed
- 8 ounces of mushrooms, chopped
- 4 Thai chilies, chopped
- 13 ounces of coconut milk
- ¼ cup of lime juice
- ¼ cup of cilantro, chopped
- A pinch of black pepper

NUTRITIONAL FACTS:

Calories: 105, Carbs: 1 g, Fat: 2 g, Protein: 15 g, Sodium: 200 mg

COOKING: 25'

PREPARATION: 10'

SERVES: 4

DIRECTIONS

1. Put the stock into a pot, bring to a simmer over medium heat, add lemongrass, ginger, and lime leaves, stir, cook for 10 minutes, strain into another pot, and heat up over medium heat again.

2. Add the chicken, mushrooms, milk, cilantro, black pepper, chilies, and lime juice, stir, simmer for 15 minutes, ladle into bowls and serve.

DINNER

SPICY COD

INGREDIENTS

- 2 pounds of cod fillets
- 1 tablespoon of flavorless oil (olive, canola, or sunflower)
- 2 cups of low sodium salsa
- 2 tablespoons of fresh chopped parsley

NUTRITIONAL FACTS:

Calories: 110, Protein: 16.5 g, Carbs: 83 g, Fat: 11 g, Sodium: 186 mg

COOKING: 30'

PREPARATION: 15'

SERVES: 4

DIRECTIONS

1. Warm the oven to 350 °F. In a large, deep baking dish, drizzle the oil along the bottom. Place the cod fillets in the dish. Pour the salsa over the fish.

2. Cover with foil for 20 minutes. Remove the foil last 10 minutes of cooking. Bake in the oven for 20–30 minutes, until the fish is flaky. Serve with white or brown rice. Garnish with parsley.

DASH DIET 2022

DAY 19

BREAKFAST

BREAKFAST FRUITS BOWLS

INGREDIENTS

- 1 cup of mango, chopped
- 1 banana, sliced
- 1 cup of pineapple, chopped
- 1 cup of almond milk

NUTRITIONAL FACTS:

Calories: 10, Carbs: 0 g, Fat: 1 g, Protein: 0 g, Sodium: 0 mg

COOKING: 0'

PREPARATION: 10'

SERVES: 2

DIRECTIONS

1. Mix the mango with the banana, pineapple, and almond milk in a bowl, stir, divide into smaller bowls, and serve.

LUNCH

FRUITED QUINOA SALAD

INGREDIENTS

- 2 cups of cooked quinoa
- 1 mango, sliced and peeled
- 1 cup of strawberry, quartered
- ½ cup of blueberries
- 2 tablespoons of pine nuts
- Chopped mint leave for garnish

Lemon vinaigrette:

- ¼ cup of olive oil
- ¼ cup of apple cider vinegar
- Zest of lemon
- 3 tablespoons of lemon juice
- 1 teaspoon of sugar

NUTRITIONAL FACTS:

Calories: 425, Carbs: 76.1 g, Proteins: 11.3 g, Fat: 10.9 g, Sodium: 16 mg

COOKING: 0'

PREPARATION: 15'

SERVES: 2

DIRECTIONS

1. For the Lemon Vinaigrette, whisk olive oil, apple cider vinegar, lemon zest and juice, and sugar to a bowl; set aside. Combine quinoa, mango strawberries, blueberries, and pine nuts in a large bowl. Stir the lemon vinaigrette and garnish it with mint. Serve and enjoy!

GRILLED PORK FAJITAS

INGREDIENTS

- ½ teaspoon of paprika
- ½ teaspoon of oregano
- ¼ teaspoon of ground coriander
- ¼ teaspoon of garlic powder
- 1 tablespoon of chili powder
- 1 pound of pork tenderloin, fat trimmed and cut into large strips
- 1 onion, sliced
- 8 whole of wheat flour tortillas, warmed
- 4 medium tomatoes, chopped
- 4 cups of shredded lettuce

NUTRITIONAL FACTS:

Calories: 250, Protein: 20 g, Carbs: 29 g, Fat: 6 g, Saturated Fat: 2 g, Sodium: 234 mg

COOKING: 15'

PREPARATION: 10'

SERVES: 8

DIRECTIONS

1. In a bowl, mix the paprika, oregano, coriander, garlic powder, and chili powder.
2. Sprinkle the spice mixture on the pork tenderloin strips and toss to coat the meat with the spices.
3. Prepare the grill and heat to 400 °F.
4. Place the meat and onion in a grill basket and broil for 20 minutes or until all sides have browned.
5. Assemble the fajitas by placing in the center of the tortillas the grilled pork and onions. Add in the tomatoes and lettuce before rolling the fajitas.

DAY 20

DASH DIET 2022

BREAKFAST

EASY VEGGIE MUFFINS

INGREDIENTS

- ¾ cup of cheddar cheese, shredded
- 1 cup of green onion, chopped
- 1 cup of tomatoes, chopped
- 1 cup of broccoli, chopped
- 2 cups of non-fat milk
- 1 cup of biscuit mix
- 4 eggs
- Cooking spray
- 1 teaspoon of Italian seasoning
- A pinch of black pepper

NUTRITIONAL FACTS:

Calories: 80, Carbs: 3 g, Fat: 5 g, Protein: 7 g, Sodium: 25 mg

COOKING: 40'

PREPARATION: 10'

SERVES: 4

DIRECTIONS

1. Grease a muffin tray with cooking spray and divide the broccoli, tomatoes, cheese, and onions in each muffin cup.

2. In a bowl, combine the green onions with milk, biscuit mix, eggs, pepper, and Italian seasoning, whisk well and pour into the muffin tray as well.

3. Cook the muffins in the oven at 375 °F for 40 minutes, divide them between plates and serve.

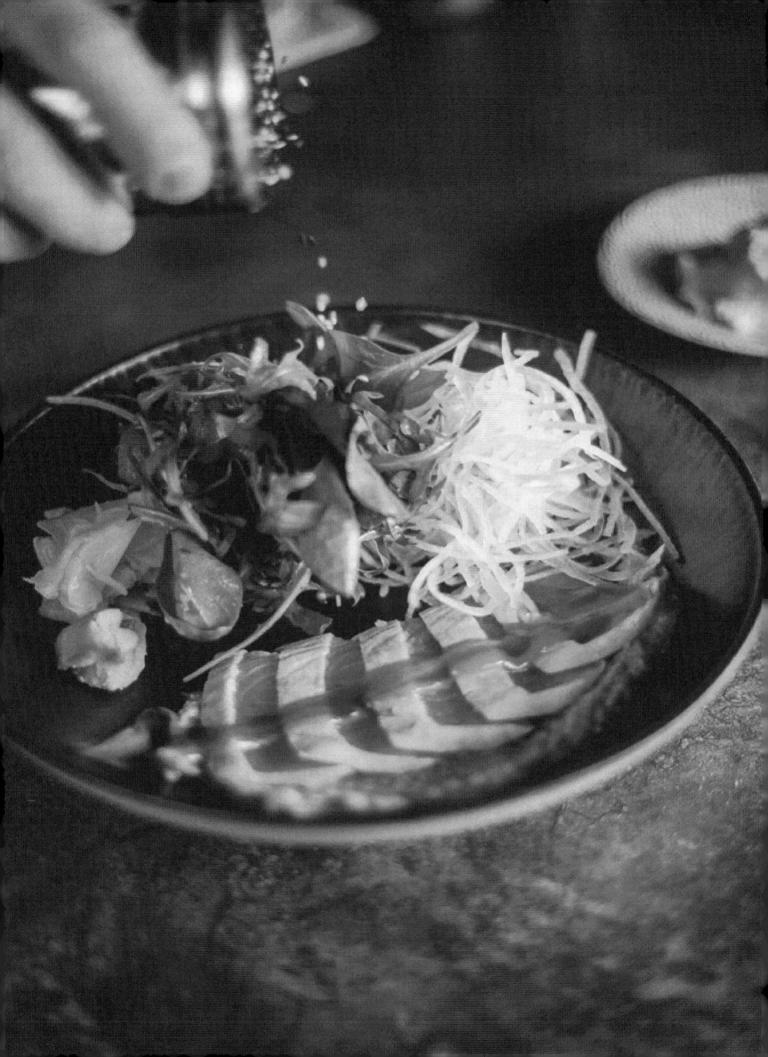

LUNCH

EASY LUNCH SALMON STEAKS

INGREDIENTS

- » 1 big salmon fillet, cut into 4 steaks
- » 3 garlic cloves, minced
- » 1 yellow onion, chopped
- » Black pepper to the taste
- » 2 tablespoons of olive oil
- » ¼ cup of parsley, chopped
- » Juice of 1 lemon
- » 1 tablespoon of thyme, chopped
- » 4 cups of water

NUTRITIONAL FACTS:

Calories: 110, Carbs: 3 g, Fat: 4 g, Protein: 15 g, Sodium 330 mg

COOKING: 20'

PREPARATION: 10'

SERVES: 4

DIRECTIONS

1. Heat a pan with the oil on medium-high heat, cook the onion and garlic within 3 minutes.

2. Add the black pepper, parsley, thyme, water, and lemon juice, stir, bring to a gentle boil, add salmon steaks, cook them for 15 minutes, drain, divide between plates and serve with a side salad for lunch.

DINNER

PROVENCE PORK MEDALLIONS

INGREDIENTS

- 1 teaspoon of Herb de Provence
- Pepper
- ½ cup of dry white wine
- 16 ounces of pork tenderloins
- Salt

NUTRITIONAL FACTS:

Calories: 105.7, Fat: 1.7 g, Carbs: 0.8 g, Protein: 22.6 g, Sugars: 0 g, Sodium: 67 mg

COOKING: 20'

PREPARATION: 10'

SERVES: 4

DIRECTIONS

1. Season the pork lightly with salt and pepper.
2. Place the pork between two pieces of parchment paper and pound with a mallet.
3. You need to have ¼ inch thick meat.
4. In a large non-stick frying pan, cook the pork over medium-high heat for 2-3 minutes per side.
5. Remove from the heat and sprinkle with herb de Provence. Remove the pork from the skillet and place it aside. Keep warm.
6. Place the skillet and overheat again. Add the wine and cook, stirring to scrape down the bits.
7. Cook until reduced slightly and pour over pork. Serve.

DAY 21

DASH DIET 2022

BREAKFAST

MUSHROOMS AND CHEESE OMELET

INGREDIENTS

- 2 tablespoons of olive oil
- A pinch of black pepper
- 3 ounces of mushrooms, sliced
- 1 cup of baby spinach, chopped
- 3 eggs, whisked
- 2 tablespoons of low-fat cheese, grated
- 1 small avocado, peeled, pitted, and cubed
- 1 tablespoon of parsley, chopped

NUTRITIONAL FACTS:

Calories: 136, Carbs: 5 g, Fat: 5 g, Protein: 16 g, Sodium: 192 mg

COOKING: 15'

PREPARATION: 10'

SERVES: 4

DIRECTIONS

1. Add the mushrooms, stir, cook them for 5 minutes and transfer to a bowl on a heated pan with the oil over medium-high heat.

2. Heat the same pan over medium-high heat, add eggs and black pepper, spread into the pan, cook within 7 minutes, and transfer to a plate.

3. Spread mushrooms, spinach, avocado, and cheese on half of the omelet, fold the other half over this mix, sprinkle parsley on top, and serve.

LUNCH

WHITE CHICKEN CHILI

INGREDIENTS

- 1 can of white chunk chicken
- 2 cans of low-sodium white beans, drained
- 1 can of low-sodium diced tomatoes
- 4 cups of low-sodium chicken broth
- 1 medium onion, chopped
- ½ medium green pepper, chopped
- 1 medium red pepper, chopped
- 2 garlic cloves, minced
- 2 teaspoons of chili powder
- 1 teaspoon of ground cumin
- 1 teaspoon of dried oregano
- Cayenne pepper, to taste
- 8 tablespoons of shredded reduced-fat Monterey Jack cheese
- 3 tablespoons of chopped fresh cilantro

NUTRITIONAL FACTS:

Calories: 225, Fat: 12.9 g, Sodium: 480 mg, Carbs: 24.7 g, Protein: 25.3 g

COOKING: 15'

PREPARATION: 20'

SERVES: 4

DIRECTIONS

1. In a soup pot, add beans, tomatoes, chicken, and chicken broth. Cover this soup pot and let it simmer over medium heat. Meanwhile, grease a nonstick pan with cooking spray. Add peppers, garlic, and onions. Sauté for 5 minutes until soft.

2. Transfer the mixture to the soup pot. Add cumin, chili powder, cayenne pepper, and oregano. Cook for 10 minutes, then garnish the chili with cilantro and 1 tablespoon cheese. Serve.

DINNER

COCONUT SHRIMP

INGREDIENTS

- ¼ cup of coconut, sweetened
- ½ teaspoon of sea salt, fine
- ¼ cup of Panko breadcrumbs
- ½ cup of coconut milk
- 12 large shrimp, peeled & deveined

NUTRITIONAL FACTS:

Calories: 249, Protein: 35 g, Fat: 1.7 g, Carbs: 1.8 g, Sodium: 79 mg, Cholesterol: 78 mg

COOKING: 15'

PREPARATION: 10'

SERVES: 4

DIRECTIONS

1. Preheat your oven to 375 °F, and then get out a baking pan. Spray it with cooking spray before setting it aside.
2. Grind your panko with coconut and salt in a food processor.
3. Add this mixture to a bowl and pour the coconut milk into another bowl.
4. Dip the shrimp in the coconut mixture and then dredge it through the panko mixture. Put the coated shrimp on the baking pan, and then bake for 15 minutes. Serve warm

CHAPTER 8

MEAL PLAN WEEK 4

DAY 22

BREAKFAST

APPLE QUINOA MUFFINS

INGREDIENTS

- ½ cup of natural, unsweetened applesauce
- 1 cup of banana, peeled and mashed
- 1 cup of quinoa
- 2 ½ cups of old-fashioned oats
- ½ cup of almond milk
- 2 tablespoons of stevia
- 1 teaspoon of vanilla extract
- 1 cup of water
- Cooking spray
- 1 teaspoon of cinnamon powder
- 1 apple, cored, peeled, and chopped

NUTRITIONAL FACTS:

Calories: 241, Carbs: 31 g, Fat: 11 g, Protein: 5 g, Sodium: 251 mg

COOKING: 35'

PREPARATION: 10'

SERVES: 4

DIRECTIONS

1. Put the water in a small pan, bring to a simmer over medium heat, add quinoa, cook within 15 minutes, fluff with a fork, and transfer to a bowl.

2. Add all the ingredients, stir, divide into a muffin pan, grease it with cooking spray, introduce in the oven, and bake within 20 minutes at 375 °F. Serve for breakfast.

LUNCH

EASY STEAMED ALASKAN COD

INGREDIENTS

- 2 tablespoons of butter
- Pepper to taste
- 1 cup of cherry tomatoes, halved
- 1 large Wild Alaskan cod filet, cut into 3 smaller pieces

NUTRITIONAL FACTS:

Calories: 132.9, Carbs: 1.9 g, Protein: 12.2 g, Fats: 8.5 g, Sodium: 296 mg

COOKING: 15'

PREPARATION: 15'

SERVES: 3

DIRECTIONS

1. In a heat-proof dish that fits inside a saucepan, add all ingredients. Cover dish with foil. Place on trivet and steam for 15 minutes. Serve and enjoy.

DINNER

SIMPLE BEEF BRISKET AND TOMATO SOUP

INGREDIENTS

- 1 tablespoon of olive oil
- 2 ½ pounds of beef brisket, trimmed of fat and cut into 8 equal parts
- A dash of ground black pepper
- 1 ½ cups of chopped onions
- 4 cloves of garlic, smashed
- 1 teaspoon of dried thyme
- 1 cup of ripe Roma tomatoes, chopped
- ¼ cup of red wine vinegar
- 1 cup of beef stock, low sodium, or homemade

NUTRITIONAL FACTS:

Calories: 229, Protein: 31 g, Carbs: 6 g, Fat: 9 g, Saturated Fat: 3 g, Sodium: 184 mg

COOKING: 3H

PREPARATION: 10'

SERVES: 8

DIRECTIONS

1. In a heavy pot, heat the oil over medium-high heat.
2. Season the brisket with ground black pepper and place in the pot.
3. Cook while constantly stirring until the beef turns brown on all sides.
4. Stir in the onions and cook until fragrant. Add in the garlic and thyme and cook for another minute until fragrant.
5. Pour in the rest of the ingredients and bring to a boil.
6. Cook until the beef is tender. This may take about 3 hours or more.

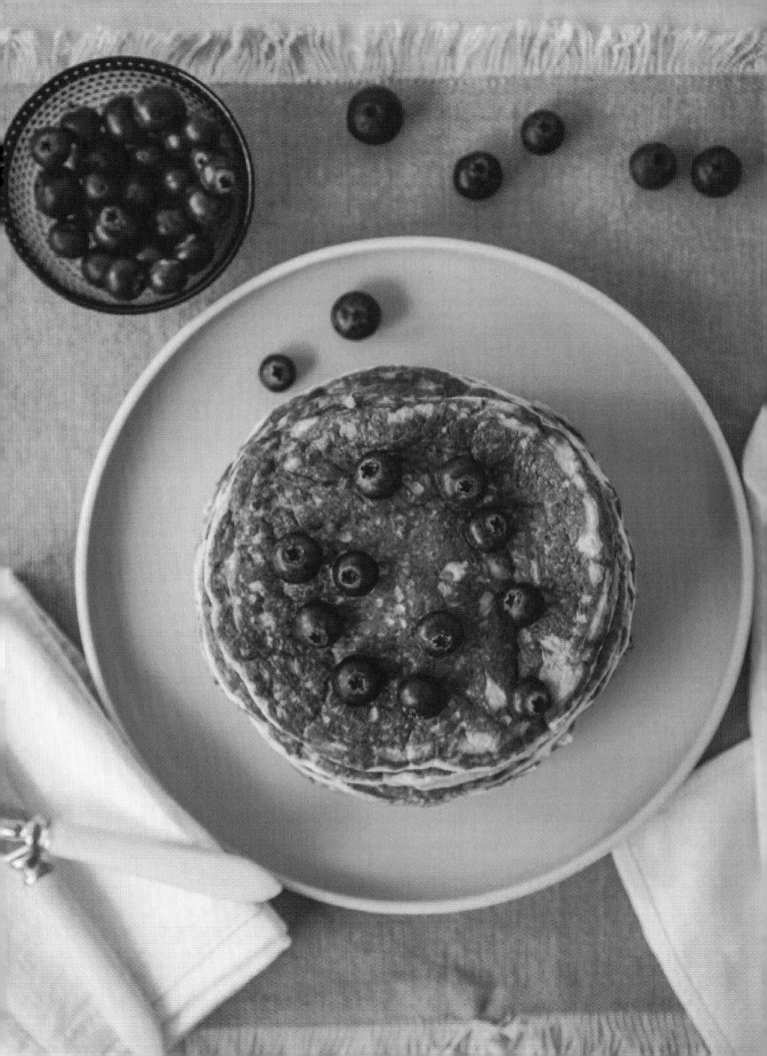

DAY 23   DASH DIET 2022

BREAKFAST

STEEL CUT OAT BLUEBERRY PANCAKES

INGREDIENTS

- 1 ½ cup of water
- ½ cup of steel-cut oats
- 1/8 teaspoon of Salt
- 1 cup of whole wheat flour
- ½ teaspoon of baking powder
- ½ teaspoon of baking soda
- 1 egg
- 1 cup of milk
- ½ cup of Greek yogurt
- 1 cup of frozen blueberries
- ¾ cup of Agave nectar

NUTRITIONAL FACTS:

Calories: 257, Protein: 14 g, Carbs: 46 g, Fat: 7 g, Sodium: 123 mg

COOKING: 15'

PREPARATION: 15'

SERVES: 4

DIRECTIONS

1. Combine your oats, salt, and water in a medium saucepan, stir, and allow to come to a boil over high heat. Adjust the heat to low, and simmer for about 10 minutes or until oats get tender. Set aside.

2. In a medium bowl, combine all your remaining ingredients, except agave nectar, then fold in oats. Preheat your skillet and lightly grease it. Cook ¼ cup of milk batter at a time for about 3 minutes per side. Garnish with Agave Nectar.

PORK AND DATES SAUCE

INGREDIENTS

- 2 tablespoons of water
- 2 tablespoons of mustard
- 1/3 cup of pitted dates
- Black pepper
- ¼ teaspoon of onion powder
- ¼ cup of coconut amino
- 1 ½ lb. of pork tenderloin
- ¼ teaspoon of smoked paprika

NUTRITIONAL FACTS:

Calories: 240, Fat: 8 g, Carbs: 13 g, Protein: 24 g, Sugars: 0 g, Sodium: 433 mg

COOKING: 40'

PREPARATION: 10'

SERVES: 6

DIRECTIONS

1. In your blender, mix the dates with water, coconut amino, mustard, paprika, pepper, and onion powder and blend well.

2. Put pork tenderloin within the roasting pan, add the dates sauce, toss to coat perfectly, introduce everything inside the oven at 400 °F, bake for 40 minutes, slice the meat, and divide it from the sauce between plates and serve.

3. Enjoy!

DINNER

FISH IN A VEGETABLE PATCH

INGREDIENTS

- 1-pound halibut fillet, skinless
- 1 tablespoon of flavorless oil (olive, canola, or sunflower)
- 1 Cup of tomato sauce
- 1 ½ tablespoon of Worcestershire sauce
- 2 large lemons, juiced
- 1 celery stick, diced
- ½ green pepper, chopped
- 1 large carrot, diced
- ½ onion, diced
- 1 lemon, sliced

NUTRITIONAL FACTS:

Calories: 80, Protein: 18.9 g, Carbs: 62 g, Fat: 9 g, Sodium: 276 mg

COOKING: 20'

PREPARATION: 15'

SERVES: 3

DIRECTIONS

1. Warm the oven to 400 °F. In a small saucepan, combine the tomato sauce, Worcestershire sauce, and lemon juice. Heat for 5 minutes.

2. In a shallow baking dish, drizzle oil along the bottom. Place the vegetables along the bottom and lay the fish over the vegetables. Pour the sauce over the fish. Cover with foil.

3. Bake fillet for 15 minutes, or until the fish is cooked and flaky. Dish out the vegetables, place the fish over the top. Garnish the fish with lemon slices. Serve with white or brown rice.

DASH DIET 2022

DAY 24

BREAKFAST

PINEAPPLE OATMEAL

INGREDIENTS

- 2 cups of old-fashioned oats
- 1 cup of walnuts, chopped
- 2 cups of pineapple, cubed
- 1 tablespoon of ginger, grated
- 2 cups of non-fat milk
- 2 eggs
- 2 tablespoons of stevia
- 2 teaspoons of vanilla extract

NUTRITIONAL FACTS:

Calories: 200, Carbs: 40 g, Fat: 1 g, Protein: 3 g, Sodium: 275 mg

COOKING: 25'

PREPARATION: 10'

SERVES: 4

DIRECTIONS

1. In a bowl, combine the oats with the pineapple, walnuts, and ginger, stir and divide into 4 ramekins.

2. Mix the milk with the eggs, stevia, and vanilla in a bowl and pour over the oats mix.

3. Bake at 400 °F within 25 minutes.

4. 4. Serve for breakfast.

LUNCH — DASH DIET 2022

SWEET POTATO-TURKEY MEATLOAF

INGREDIENTS

- 1 large sweet potato, peeled and cubed
- 1 pound ground turkey (breast)
- 1 large egg
- 1 small sweet onion, finely chopped
- 2 cloves of garlic, minced
- 2 slices whole-wheat breadcrumbs
- ¼ cup of honey barbecue sauce
- ¼ cup of ketchup
- 2 tablespoons of Dijon mustard
- 1 tablespoon of fresh ground pepper
- ½ tablespoon of salt

NUTRITIONAL FACTS:

Calories: 133, Protein: 85 g, Carbs: 50 g, Fat: 34 g, Sodium: 202 mg

COOKING: 25'

PREPARATION: 15'

SERVES: 4

DIRECTIONS

1. Warm the oven to 350 °F. Grease a baking dish. In a large pot, boil a cup of lightly salted water, add the sweet potato. Cook until tender. Drain the water. Mash the potato.

2. Mix the honey barbecue sauce, ketchup, and Dijon mustard in a small bowl. Mix thoroughly. In a large bowl, mix the turkey and the egg. Add the sweet onion, garlic. Pour in the combined sauces. Add the bread crumbs. Season the mixture with salt and pepper.

3. Add the sweet potato. Combine thoroughly with your hands. If the mixture feels wet, add more breadcrumbs. Shape the mixture into a loaf. Place in the loaf pan. Bake for 25–35 minutes until the meat is cooked through. Broil for 5 minutes. Slice and serve.

DINNER

STEAMED BLUE CRABS

INGREDIENTS

- 30 live blue crabs
- ½ cup of seafood seasoning
- ¼ cup of salt
- 3 cups of beer
- 3 cups of distilled white vinegar

NUTRITIONAL FACTS:

Calories: 77, Protein: 9.8 g, Carbs: 31 g, Fat: 7 g, Sodium: 119 mg

COOKING: 10'

PREPARATION: 15'

SERVES: 6

DIRECTIONS

1. In a large stockpot, combine the seasoning, salt, beer, and white vinegar. Bring it to a boil. Put each crab upside down, then stick a knife into the shell just before cooking them. Cover the lid, leaving a crack for the steam to vent.

2. Steam the crabs until they turn bright orange and float to the top. Allow them to cook for another 2 - 3 minutes. Serve immediately.

DAY 25 — DASH DIET 2022

BREAKFAST

BANANA & CINNAMON OATMEAL

INGREDIENTS

- 2 cups of quick-cooking oats
- 4 cups of fat-free milk
- 1 teaspoon of ground cinnamon
- 2 chopped large ripe banana
- 4 teaspoons of brown sugar
- Extra ground cinnamon

NUTRITIONAL FACTS:

Calories: 215, Fat: 2 g, Carbs: 42 g, Protein: 10 g, Sugars: 1 g, Sodium: 40 mg

COOKING: 0'

PREPARATION: 5'

SERVES: 6

DIRECTIONS

1. Place the milk in a skillet and bring to boil. Add the oats and cook over medium heat until thickened, for 2 to 4 minutes.

2. Stir intermittently. Add the cinnamon, brown sugar, and banana and stir to combine. If you want, serve with the extra cinnamon and milk. Enjoy!

LUNCH

TURKEY WRAP

INGREDIENTS

- 2 slices of low-fat Turkey breast (deli-style)
- 4 tablespoons of non-fat cream cheese
- ½ cup of lettuce leaves
- ½ cup of carrots, slice into a stick
- 2 homemade wraps or store-bought whole-wheat tortilla wrap

NUTRITIONAL FACTS:

Calories: 224, Carbs: 35 g, Protein: 10.3 g, Fat: 3.8 g, Sodium: 293 mg

COOKING: 10'

PREPARATION: 15'

SERVES: 2

DIRECTIONS

1. Prepare all the ingredients. Spread 2 tablespoons of non-fat cream cheese on each wrap. Arrange lettuce leaves, then add a slice of turkey breast; a slice of carrots stick on top. Roll and cut it in half. Serve and enjoy!

DINNER

ASIAN SALMON

INGREDIENTS

- 1 cup of fresh fruit, diced
- ¼ teaspoon of Black Pepper
- 2 Salmon fillets, 4 ounces of each
- ¼ teaspoon of Sesame oil
- 1 teaspoon of Soy Sauce, low sodium
- 2 cloves garlic, minced
- ½ cup of pineapple Juice, sugar-free

NUTRITIONAL FACTS:

Calories: 247, Protein: 27 g, Fat: 7 g, Carbs: 19 g, Sodium: 350 mg, Cholesterol: 120 mg

COOKING: 20'

PREPARATION: 10'

SERVES: 2

DIRECTIONS

1. Start by getting out a bowl and mixing your garlic, soy sauce, ginger, and pineapple juice. Place your fish in the dough and make sure it's covered. It marinates for an hour.

2. Flip the fillets after thirty minutes, and then heat the oven to 375 °F.

3. Get out aluminum squares and grease them with cooking spray. Put the salmon fillet on each square, and drizzle with pepper, diced fruit and sesame oil. Fold the aluminum sheet to seal the fish, and then place them on the baking sheet.

4. Bake for ten minutes per side before serving.

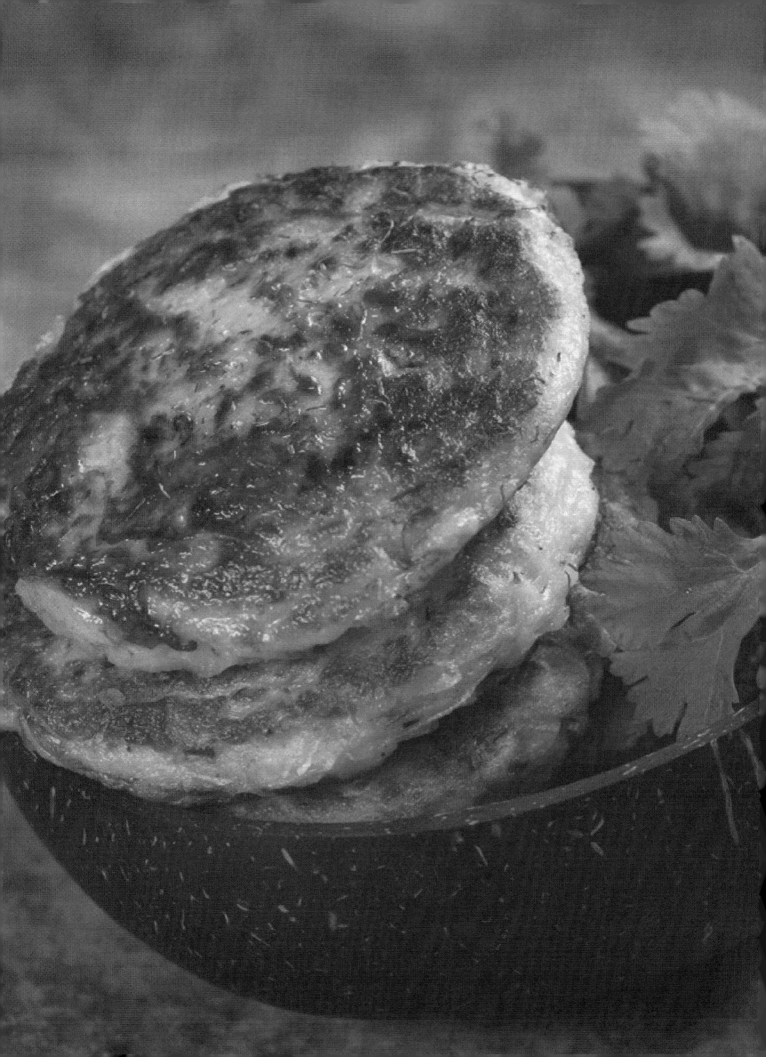

DAY 26

BREAKFAST

ZUCCHINI PANCAKES

INGREDIENTS

- 4 large zucchinis
- 4 green onions, diced
- 1/3 cup of milk
- 1 organic egg
- Sea Salt, just a pinch
- Black pepper, grated
- 2 tablespoons of olive oil

NUTRITIONAL FACTS:

Calories: 70, Carbs: 8 g, Fat: 3 g, Protein: 2 g, Cholesterol: 43 mg, Sodium: 60 mg, Potassium: 914 mg

COOKING: 10'

PREPARATION: 15'

SERVES: 4

DIRECTIONS

1. First, wash the zucchinis and grate them with a cheese grater. Mix the egg and add in the grated zucchinis and milk in a large bowl. Warm oil in a skillet and sauté onions in it.

2. Put the egg batter into the skillet and make pancakes. Once cooked from both sides. Serve by sprinkling salt and pepper on top..

LUNCH

WHITE BEANS STEW

INGREDIENTS

- 1 cup of white beans, soaked
- 1 cup of low-sodium vegetable broth
- 1 cup of zucchini, chopped
- 1 teaspoon of tomato paste
- 1 tablespoon of avocado oil
- 4 cups of water
- ½ teaspoon of peppercorns
- ½ teaspoon of ground black pepper
- ¼ teaspoon of ground nutmeg

NUTRITIONAL FACTS:

Calories: 184, Protein: 12.3 g, Carbs: 32.6 g, Fat: 1 g, Sodium: 55 mg

COOKING: 55'

PREPARATION: 15'

SERVES: 4

DIRECTIONS

1. Heat avocado oil in the saucepan, add zucchinis and roast them for 5 minutes. After this, add white beans, vegetable broth, tomato paste, water, peppercorns, ground black pepper, and ground nutmeg. Simmer the stew within 50 minutes on low heat.

DINNER

GARLIC PEPPER CHICKEN

INGREDIENTS

- 2 chicken breasts, cut into strips
- 2 bell peppers, cut into strips
- 5 garlic cloves, chopped
- 3 tablespoons of water
- 2 tablespoons of olive oil
- 1 tablespoon of paprika
- 2 teaspoons of black pepper
- ½ teaspoon of salt

NUTRITIONAL FACTS:

Calories: 462, Fat: 25.7 g, Protein: 44.7 g, Carbs: 14.8 g, Sodium 720 mg

COOKING: 15'

PREPARATION: 15'

SERVES: 4

DIRECTIONS

1. Warm the olive oil in a large saucepan over medium heat. Add garlic and sauté for 2-3 minutes. Add the peppers and cook for 3 minutes. Add the chicken and spices and stir to coat. Add the water and stir well. Bring to boil. Cover and simmer for 10-15 minutes. Serve and enjoy.

DASH DIET 2022

DAY 27

BREAKFAST

CARROT CAKE OVERNIGHT OATS

INGREDIENTS

- ½ cup of rolled oats
- ½ cup of plain nonfat or low-fat Greek yogurt
- ½ cup of nonfat or low-fat milk
- ¼ cup of shredded carrot
- 2 tablespoons of raisins
- ½ teaspoon of ground cinnamon
- 1 to 2 tablespoons of chopped walnuts (optional)

NUTRITIONAL FACTS:

Calories: 331, Fat: 3 g, Sodium: 141 mg, Carbs: 59 g, Fiber: 8 g, Sugars: 26 g, Protein: 22 g

COOKING: 2'

PREPARATION: OVERNIGHT

SERVES: 1

DIRECTIONS

1. Mix all of the ingredients in a lidded jar, shake well, and refrigerate overnight. Serve.

LUNCH

SPICY TOFU BURRITO BOWLS WITH CILANTRO AVOCADO SAUCE

INGREDIENTS

For the sauce:

- ¼ cup of plain nonfat Greek yogurt
- ½ cup of fresh cilantro leaves
- ½ ripe avocado, peeled
- Zest and juice of 1 lime
- 2 garlic cloves, peeled
- ¼ teaspoon of kosher or sea salt
- 2 tablespoons of water

For the burrito bowls:

- 1 (14 ounces) package extra-firm tofu
- 1 tablespoon of canola oil
- 1 yellow or orange bell pepper, diced
- 2 tablespoons of taco seasoning
- ¼ teaspoon of kosher or sea salt
- 2 cups of Fluffy Brown rice
- 1 (15 ounces) can black beans, drained

NUTRITIONAL FACTS:

Calories: 383, Fat: 13 g, Sodium: 438 mg, Carbs: 48 g, Protein: 21 g

COOKING: 15'

PREPARATION: 15'

SERVES: 4

DIRECTIONS

1. Place all the sauce ingredients in the bowl of a food processor or blender and purée until smooth. Taste and adjust the seasoning, if necessary. Refrigerate until ready for use.

2. Put the tofu on your plate lined with a kitchen towel. Put another kitchen towel over the tofu and place a heavy pot on top, changing towels if they become soaked. Let it stand within 15 minutes to remove the moisture. Cut the tofu into 1-inch cubes.

3. Warm the canola oil in a large skillet over medium heat. Add the tofu and bell pepper, and sauté, breaking up the tofu into smaller pieces for 4 to 5 minutes. Stir in the taco seasoning, salt, and ¼ cup of water. Evenly divide the rice and black beans among 4 bowls. Top with the tofu/bell pepper mixture and top with the cilantro avocado sauce.

DINNER

BAKED CHICKEN

INGREDIENTS

- 2 lbs. of chicken tenders
- 1 large zucchini
- 1 cup of grape tomatoes
- 2 tablespoons of olive oil
- 3 dill sprigs

For topping:

- 2 tablespoons of feta cheese, crumbled
- 1 tablespoon of olive oil
- 1 tablespoon of fresh lemon juice
- 1 tablespoon of fresh dill, chopped

NUTRITIONAL FACTS:

Calories: 557, Fat: 28.6 g, Protein: 67.9 g, Carbs: 5.2 g, Sodium: 760 mg

COOKING: 35'

PREPARATION: 15'

SERVES: 4

DIRECTIONS

1. Warm the oven to 200 °C/ 400 °F. Drizzle the olive oil on a baking tray, then place chicken, zucchini, dill, and tomatoes on the tray. Season with salt. Bake chicken within 30 minutes.

2. Meanwhile, in a small bowl, stir all topping ingredients. Place chicken on the serving tray, then top with veggies and discard dill sprigs. Sprinkle topping mixture on top of chicken and vegetables. Serve and enjoy.

DAY 28

DASH DIET 2022

BREAKFAST

EGG WHITE BREAKFAST MIX

INGREDIENTS

- 1 yellow onion, chopped
- 3 plum tomatoes, chopped
- 10 ounces of spinach, chopped
- A pinch of black pepper
- 2 tablespoons of water
- 12 egg whites
- Cooking spray

NUTRITIONAL FACTS:

Calories: 31, Carbs: 0 g, Fat: 2 g, Protein: 3 g, Sodium: 55 mg

COOKING: 10'

PREPARATION: 10'

SERVES: 4

DIRECTIONS

1. Mix the egg whites with water and pepper in a bowl. Grease a pan with cooking spray, heat up over medium heat, add ¼ of the egg whites, spread into the pan, and cook for 2 minutes.

2. Spoon ¼ of the spinach, tomatoes, and onion, fold and add to a plate. 4. Serve for breakfast. Enjoy!

LUNCH

CHICKEN WITH POTATOES OLIVES & SPROUTS

INGREDIENTS

- 1 lb. of chicken breasts, skinless, boneless, and cut into pieces
- ¼ cup of olives, quartered
- 1 teaspoon of oregano
- 1 ½ teaspoon of Dijon mustard
- 1 lemon juice
- 1/3 cup of vinaigrette dressing
- 1 medium onion, diced
- 3 cups of potatoes cut into pieces
- 4 cups of Brussels sprouts, trimmed and quartered
- ¼ teaspoon of pepper
- ¼ teaspoon of salt

NUTRITIONAL FACTS:

Calories: 397, Fat: 13 g, Protein: 38.3 g, Carbs: 31.4 g, Sodium: 175 mg

COOKING: 35'

PREPARATION: 15'

SERVES: 4

DIRECTIONS

1. Warm the oven to 400 °F. Place chicken in the center of the baking tray, then place the potatoes, sprouts, and onions around the chicken.

2. Mix the vinaigrette, oregano, mustard, lemon juice, and salt in a small bowl, and pour over the chicken and veggies. Sprinkle olives and season with pepper.

3. Bake in preheated oven for 20 minutes. Transfer chicken to a plate. Stir the vegetables and roast for 15 minutes more. Serve and enjoy.

DINNER

GINGER SESAME SALMON

INGREDIENTS

- 4 ounces of salmon
- ¼ cup of low-sodium soy sauce
- 2 tablespoons of Balsamic vinegar
- ½ teaspoon of sesame oil
- 2-inch chunk ginger, peeled and grated
- 1 garlic clove, minced
- 1 teaspoon of flavorless oil (olive, canola, or sunflower)
- 1 teaspoon of sesame seeds
- 1 teaspoon of green onion, minced

NUTRITIONAL FACTS:

Calories: 422, Protein: 10.8 g, Carbs: 5.7 g, Fat: 18 g, Sodium: 300 mg

COOKING: 5'

PREPARATION: 15'

SERVES: 2

DIRECTIONS

1. Combine the soy sauce, balsamic vinegar, sesame oil, garlic, and ginger in a glass dish. Place the salmon in the dish. Cover, marinate for 15-60 minutes in the fridge.

2. In a nonstick skillet, heat 1 teaspoon of oil. Sauté the fish until it becomes firm and golden on each side. Sprinkle the sesame seeds in the pan. Heat for 1 minute. Serve immediately. Garnish with green onion.

CONCLUSION

Statistics have it that one in three people have hypertension in America, and those that have normal blood pressure at the age of 50 or so have a 90% chance of getting affected in the near future. This is a high number considering how dangerous to your health hypertension can be. Having hypertension also means that you are prone to other health-related illnesses and diseases, which means an unhealthy life, and sometimes short life.

This is not something that you cannot avoid, though, because making the right dietary choices has been seen to work really well to improve people's health and reduce the chances of suffering from hypertension and other health-related issues. The right choices can also make the existing condition manageable, and you can still enjoy a longer, healthier life after that.

It is not too late to venture into a DASH Diet, a diet plan that will bring significant changes in your health and life in general. This, coupled with staying active, limiting alcohol consumption, controlling your body weight, and staying stress-free, will help you enjoy a long, happy life.

DASH diet is effortless to follow as it is the most accessible diet plan, but if you have to make substantial diet changes. In order to fully adopt the DASH diet in your life, it is good to start making small changes bit by bit. Replace some of the unhealthy foods with healthy foods one day at a time. It will not be hard to stick to the diet plan this way. Convince your mind that healthy foods are the right foods to eat at all times and always have these healthy foods at your disposal in the place of unhealthy ones.

KEEP COOKING TASTY AND HEALTHY RECIPES AFTER YOU FINISH YOUR MEAL PLAN, MORE THAN 99 RECIPES AT YOUR DISPOSAL SO YOU CAN INDULGE YOURSELF AND HAVE FUN WITH YOUR WHOLE FAMILY!

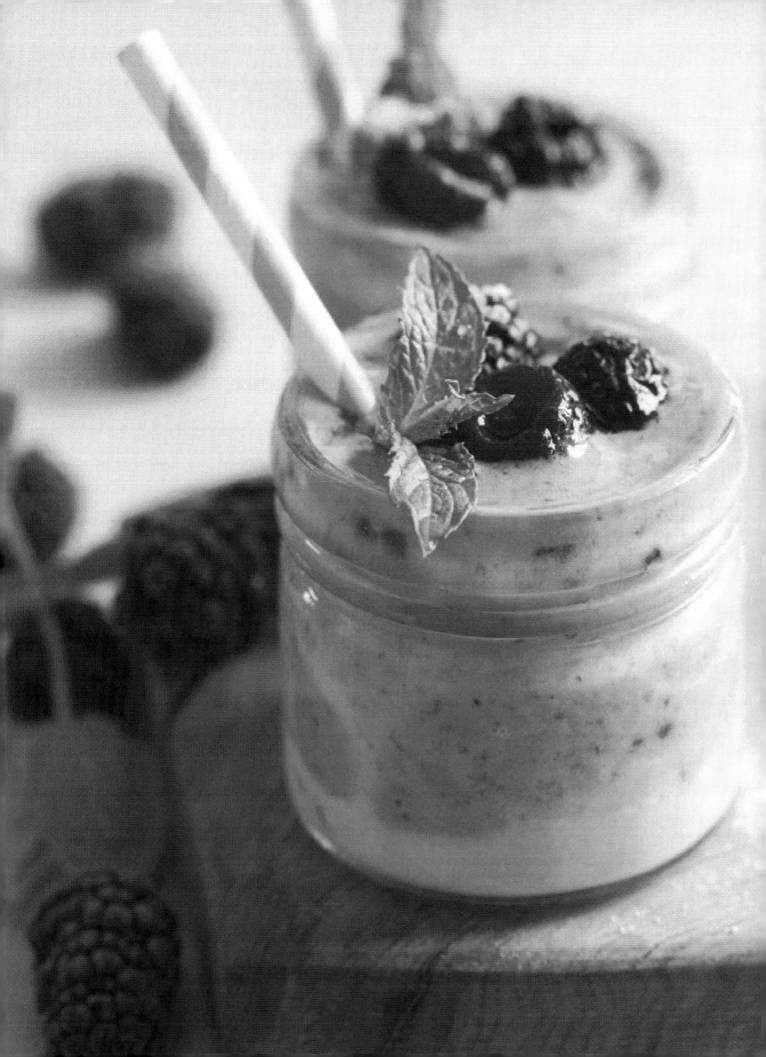

CHAPTER 9
SMOOTHIE RECIPES

1. CREAMY APPLE-AVOCADO SMOOTHIE

INGREDIENTS

- ½ medium avocado, peeled and pitted
- 1 medium apple, chopped
- 1 cup baby spinach leaves
- 1 cup nonfat vanilla Greek yogurt
- ½ to 1 cup of water
- 1 cup ice
- 1 freshly squeezed lemon juice (optional)

NUTRITIONAL FACTS:

Calories: 200, Fat: 7 g, Sodium: 56 mg, Potassium: 378 mg, Carbs: 27 g, Fiber: 5 g, Sugars: 20 g, Protein: 10 g

COOKING: 0'

PREPARATION: 15'

SERVES: 2

DIRECTIONS

1. Blend all of the fixing using a blender, and blend until smooth and creamy. Put a squeeze of lemon juice on top if desired, and serve immediately.

2. STRAWBERRY, ORANGE, AND BEET SMOOTHIE

INGREDIENTS

- 1 cup nonfat milk
- 1 cup of frozen strawberries
- 1 medium beet, cooked, peeled, and cubed
- 1 orange, peeled and quartered
- 1 frozen banana, peeled and chopped
- 1 cup nonfat vanilla Greek yogurt
- 1 cup ice

NUTRITIONAL FACTS:

Calories: 266, Fat: 0 g, Cholesterol: 7 mg, Sodium: 104 mg, Carbohydrates: 51 g, Fiber: 6 g, Sugars: 34 g, Protein: 15 g

COOKING: 0'

PREPARATION: 5'

SERVES: 2

DIRECTIONS

1. In a blender, combine all of the fixings, and blend until smooth. Serve immediately.

3. MIXED BERRIES SMOOTHIE

INGREDIENTS

- ¼ cup frozen blueberries
- ¼ cup frozen blackberries
- 1 cup unsweetened almond milk
- 1 teaspoon vanilla bean extract
- 3 teaspoons flaxseeds
- 1 scoop chilled Greek yogurt
- Stevia as needed

NUTRITIONAL FACTS:

Calories: 221, Fat: 9 g, Protein: 21 g, Carbs: 10 g, Sodium: 78 m g

COOKING: 0'

PREPARATION: 4'

SERVES: 2

DIRECTIONS

1. Mix everything in a blender and emulsify.
2. Pulse the mixture four time until you have your desired thickness.
3. Pour the mixture into a glass and enjoy!

4. SATISFYING BERRY AND ALMOND SMOOTHIE

INGREDIENTS

- 1 cup blueberries, frozen
- 1 whole banana
- ½ cup almond milk
- 1 tablespoon almond butter
- Water as needed

NUTRITIONAL FACTS:

Calories: 321, Fat: 11 g, Carbs: 55 g, Protein: 5 g, Sodium: 46 mg

COOKING: 0'

PREPARATION: 10'

SERVES: 4

DIRECTIONS

1. Add the listed ingredients to your blender and blend well until you have a smoothie-like texture.
2. Chill and serve.
3. Enjoy!

5. REFRESHING MANGO AND PEAR SMOOTHIE

INGREDIENTS

- 1 ripe mango, cored and chopped
- ½ mango, peeled, pitted and chopped
- 1 cup kale, chopped
- ½ cup plain Greek yogurt
- 2 ice cubes

NUTRITIONAL FACTS:

Calories: 293, Fat: 8 g, Carbs: 53 g, Protein: 8 g, Sodium: 36 mg

COOKING: 0'

PREPARATION: 10'

SERVES: 1

DIRECTIONS

1. Add pear, mango, yogurt, kale, and mango to a blender and puree.
2. Add ice and blend until you have a smooth texture.
3. Serve and enjoy!

6. BLACKBERRY AND APPLE SMOOTHIE

INGREDIENTS

- 2 cups frozen blackberries
- ½ cup apple cider
- 1 apple, cubed
- 2/3 cup non-fat lemon yogurt

NUTRITIONAL FACTS:

Calories: 200, Fat: 10 g, Carbs: 14 g, Protein: 2 g, Sodium: 42 mg

COOKING: 20'

PREPARATION: 5'

SERVES: 5

DIRECTIONS

1. Add the listed ingredients to your blender and blend until smooth.
2. Serve chilled!

7. MINT FLAVORED PEAR SMOOTHIE

INGREDIENTS

- ¼ honey dew
- 2 green pears, ripe
- ½ apple, juiced
- 1 cup ice cubes
- ½ cup fresh mint leaves

NUTRITIONAL FACTS:

Calories: 200, Fat: 10 g, Carbs: 14 g, Protein: 2g, Sodium: 63 mg

COOKING: 5'

PREPARATION: 5'

SERVES: 2

DIRECTIONS

1. Add the listed ingredients to your blender and blend until smooth.
2. Serve chilled!

8. CHILLED WATERMELON SMOOTHIE

INGREDIENTS

- 1 cup watermelon chunks
- ½ cup coconut water
- 1 ½ teaspoons lime juice
- 4 mint leaves
- 4 ice cubes

NUTRITIONAL FACTS:

Calories: 200, Fat: 10 g, Carbs: 14 g, Protein: 2 g, Sodium: 40 mg

COOKING: 10'

PREPARATION: 5'

SERVES: 2

DIRECTIONS

1. Add the listed ingredients to your blender and blend until smooth.
2. Serve chilled!

9. BLUEBERRY-VANILLA YOGURT SMOOTHIE

INGREDIENTS

- 1½ cups frozen blueberries
- 1 cup nonfat vanilla Greek yogurt
- 1 frozen banana, peeled and sliced
- ½ cup nonfat or low-fat milk
- 1 cup ice

NUTRITIONAL FACTS:

Calories: 228, Fat: 1 g, Sodium: 63 mg, Potassium: 470 mg, Carbs: 45 g, Fiber: 5 g, Sugars: 34 g, Protein: 12 g

COOKING: 0'

PREPARATION: 5'

SERVES: 2

DIRECTIONS

1. In a blender, combine all of the fixing listed, and blend until smooth and creamy. Serve immediately.

10. BANANA-PEANUT BUTTER AND GREENS SMOOTHIE

INGREDIENTS

- 1 c. chopped and packed Romaine lettuce
- 1 frozen medium banana
- 1 tbsp. all-natural peanut butter
- 1 c. cold almond milk

NUTRITIONAL FACTS:

Calories: 349.3, Fat: 9.7 g, Carbs: 57.4 g, Protein: 8.1 g, Sugars: 4.3 g, Sodium: 18 mg

COOKING: 0'

PREPARATION: 5'

SERVES: 1

DIRECTIONS

1. In a heavy-duty blender, add all ingredients. Puree until smooth and creamy. Serve and enjoy.

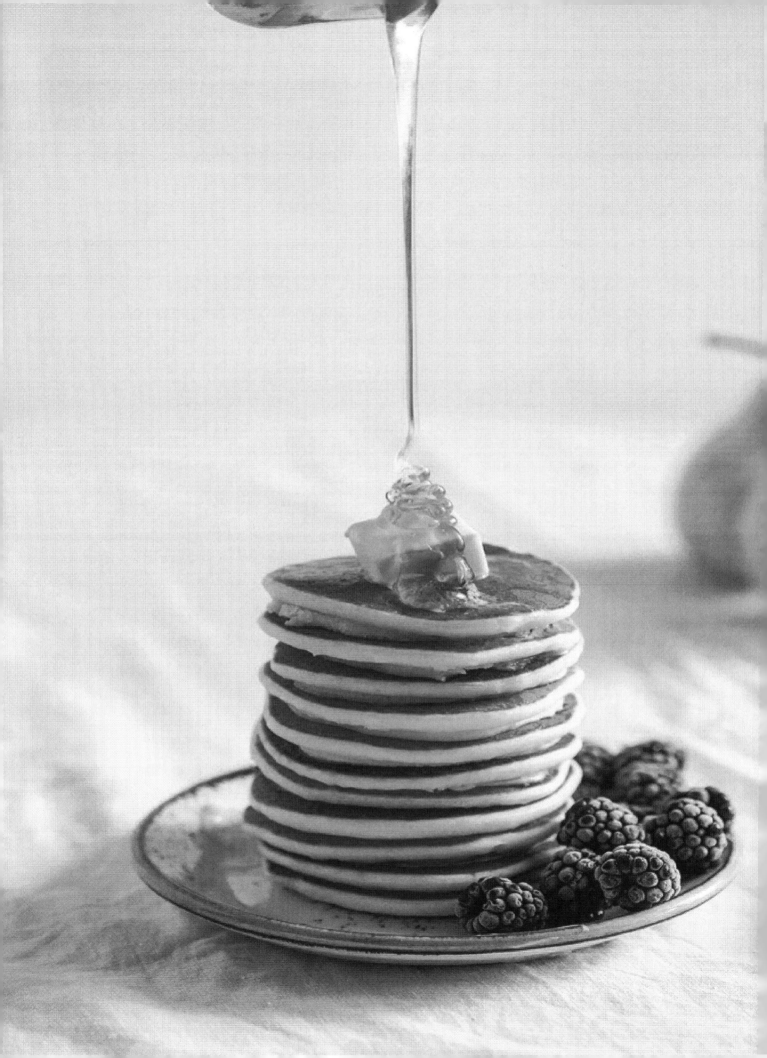

CHAPTER 10

SMOOTHIE RECIPES

11. VERY BERRY MUESLI

INGREDIENTS

- 1 c. Oats
- 1 c. Fruit flavored Yogurt
- ½ c. Milk
- 1/8 tsp. Salt
- ½ c dried Raisins
- ½ c. Chopped Apple
- ½ c. Frozen Blueberries
- ¼ c. chopped Walnuts

NUTRITIONAL FACTS:

Calories: 195, Protein: 6 g, -Carbs: 31 g, Fat: 4 g, Sodium: 0 mg

COOKING: 0'

PREPARATION: 15'

SERVES: 2

DIRECTIONS

1. Combine your yogurt, salt, and oats in a medium bowl, mix well, and then cover it tightly. Fridge for at least 6 hours. Add your raisins and apples the gently fold. Top with walnuts and serve. Enjoy!

12. SWEET POTATO TOAST THREE WAYS

INGREDIENTS

- 1 large sweet potato, unpeeled
- Topping Choice #1:
- 4 tablespoons peanut butter
- 1 ripe banana, sliced
- Dash ground cinnamon
- Topping Choice #2:
- ½ avocado, peeled, pitted, and mashed
- 2 eggs (1 per slice)
- Topping Choice #3:
- 4 tablespoons nonfat or low-fat ricotta cheese
- 1 tomato, sliced
- Dash black pepper

NUTRITIONAL FACTS:

Calories: 137, Fat: 0 g, Sodium: 17 mg, Potassium: 265 mg, Carbs: 32 g, Fiber: 4 g, Sugars: 0 g, Protein: 2 g

COOKING: 25'

PREPARATION: 15'

SERVES: 2

DIRECTIONS

1. Slice the sweet potato lengthwise into ¼-inch thick slices. Place the sweet potato slices in a toaster on high for about 5 minutes or until cooked through.

2. Repeat multiple times, if necessary, depending on your toaster settings. Top with your desired topping choices and enjoy.

13. STEEL-CUT OATMEAL WITH PLUMS AND PEAR

INGREDIENTS

- 2 cups of water
- 1 cup nonfat or low-fat milk
- 1 cup steel-cut oats
- 1 cup dried plums, chopped
- 1 medium pear, cored, and skin removed, diced
- 4 tablespoons almonds, roughly chopped

NUTRITIONAL FACTS:

Calories: 307, Fat: 6 g, Sodium: 132 mg, Potassium: 640 mg, Carbs: 58 g, Fiber: 9 g, Sugars: 24 g, Protein: 9 g

COOKING: 25'

PREPARATION: 15'

SERVES: 4

DIRECTIONS

1. Mix the water, milk, plus oats in a medium pot and bring to a boil over high heat. Reduce the heat and cover. Simmer for about 10 minutes, stirring occasionally.

2. Add the plums and pear, and cover. Simmer for another 10 minutes. Turn off the heat and let stand within 5 minutes until all of the liquid is absorbed. To serve, top each portion with a sprinkling of almonds.

14. FRENCH TOAST WITH APPLESAUCE

INGREDIENTS

- ¼ c. unsweetened applesauce
- ½ c. skim milk
- 2 packets Stevia
- 2 eggs
- 6 slices whole-wheat bread
- 1 tsp. ground cinnamon

NUTRITIONAL FACTS:

Calories: 122.6, Fat: 2.6 g, Carbs: 18.3 g, Protein: 6.5 g, Sugars: 14.8 g, Sodium: 11 mg

COOKING: 5'

PREPARATION: 5'

SERVES: 6

DIRECTIONS

1. Put the applesauce, sugar, cinnamon, milk, and eggs in a bowl and mix them well. Soak the bread into the applesauce mixture until wet. Heat a large nonstick skillet on medium fire.

2. Put soaked bread on one side and another on the other side. Cook in a single layer within 2-3 minutes per side on medium-low fire or until lightly browned. Serve and enjoy.

15. BREAKFAST HASH

INGREDIENTS

- Nonstick cooking spray
- 2 large sweet potatoes, ½-inch cubes
- 1 scallion, finely chopped
- ¼ teaspoon salt
- ½ teaspoon freshly ground black pepper
- 8 ounces extra-lean ground beef (96% or leaner)
- 1 medium onion, diced
- 2 garlic cloves, minced
- 1 red bell pepper, diced
- ¼ teaspoon ground cumin
- ¼ teaspoon paprika
- 2 cups coarsely chopped kale leaves
- ¾ cup shredded reduced-fat Cheddar cheese
- 4 large eggs

NUTRITIONAL FACTS:

Calories: 323, Fat: 15 g, Carbs: 23 g, Fiber: 4 g, Protein: 25 g, Potassium: 676 mg, Sodium: 587 mg

COOKING: 25'

PREPARATION: 15'

SERVES: 4

DIRECTIONS

1. Oiled a large skillet with cooking spray and heat over medium heat. Add the sweet potatoes, scallion, salt, and pepper. Sauté for 10 minutes, stirring often.

2. Add the beef, onion, garlic, bell pepper, cumin, and paprika. Sauté, frequently stirring, for about 4 minutes, or until the meat browns. Add the kale to the skillet and stir until wilted. Sprinkle with the Cheddar cheese.

3. Make four wells in the hash batter and crack an egg into each. Cover and let the eggs cook until the white is fully cooked and the yolk is to your liking. Divide into 4 storage containers

16. CHIA SEEDS BREAKFAST MIX

INGREDIENTS

- 2 cups old-fashioned oats
- 4 tablespoons chia seeds
- 4 tablespoons coconut sugar
- 3 cups of coconut milk
- 1 teaspoon lemon zest, grated
- 1 cup blueberries

NUTRITIONAL FACTS:

Calories: 69, Carbs: 0 g, Fat: 5 g, Protein: 3 g, Sodium: 0 mg

COOKING: 0'

PREPARATION: 8H

SERVES: 4

DIRECTIONS

1. In a bowl, mix the oats with chia seeds, sugar, milk, lemon zest, and blueberries. Stir the mixture, divide into cups and keep in the fridge for 8 hours. 2. Serve for breakfast.

17. BREAKFAST FRUITS BOWLS

INGREDIENTS

- 1 cup mango, chopped
- 1 banana, sliced
- 1 cup pineapple, chopped
- 1 cup almond milk

NUTRITIONAL FACTS:

Calories: 10, Carbs: 0 g, Fat: 1 g, Protein: 0 g, Sodium: 0 mg

COOKING: 0'

PREPARATION: 10'

SERVES: 2

DIRECTIONS

1. Mix the mango with the banana, pineapple, and almond milk in a bowl, stir, divide into smaller bowls, and serve.

18. PUMPKIN COOKIES

INGREDIENTS

- 2 cups whole wheat flour
- 1 cup old-fashioned oats
- 1 teaspoon baking soda
- 1 teaspoon pumpkin pie spice
- 15 ounces pumpkin puree
- 1 cup coconut oil, melted
- 1 cup of coconut sugar
- 1 egg
- ½ cup pepitas, roasted
- ½ cup cherries, dried

NUTRITIONAL FACTS:

Calories: 150, Carbs: 24 g, Fat: 8g, Protein: 1 g, Sodium: 220 mg

COOKING: 25'

PREPARATION: 10'

SERVES: 6

DIRECTIONS

1. Mix the flour the oats, baking soda, pumpkin spice, pumpkin puree, oil, sugar, egg, pepitas, and cherries in a bowl, stir well, shape medium cookies out of this mix, arrange them all on a baking sheet, then bake within 25 minutes at 350 degrees F. Serve the cookies for breakfast.

19. VEGGIE SCRAMBLE

INGREDIENTS

- 1 egg
- 1 tablespoon water
- ¼ cup broccoli, chopped
- ¼ cup mushrooms, chopped
- A pinch of black pepper
- 1 tablespoon low-fat mozzarella, shredded
- 1 tablespoon walnuts, chopped
- Cooking spray

NUTRITIONAL FACTS:

Calories: 128, Carbs: 24 g, Fat: 0 g, Protein: 9 g, Sodium: 86 mg

COOKING: 2'

PREPARATION: 10'

SERVES: 1

DIRECTIONS

1. Put some cooking spray on a ramekin, add the egg, water, pepper, mushrooms, and broccoli, and mix well.
2. Put the ramekin in the microwave and cook for 2 minutes. Add mozzarella and walnuts on top and serve for breakfast.

20. PESTO OMELET

INGREDIENTS

- 2 teaspoons olive oil
- Handful cherry tomatoes, chopped
- 3 tablespoons pistachio pesto
- A pinch of black pepper
- 4 eggs

NUTRITIONAL FACTS:

Calories: 240, Carbs: 23 g, Fat: 9 g, Protein: 17 g, Sodium: 292 mg

COOKING: 6'

PREPARATION: 10'

SERVES: 2

DIRECTIONS

1. In a bowl, combine the eggs with cherry tomatoes, black pepper, and pistachio pesto and mix well. Add eggs mix, spread into the pan, cook for 3 minutes, flip, cook for 3 minutes more, divide between 2 plates, and serve on a heated pan with the oil over medium-high heat.

21. BAGELS MADE HEALTHY

INGREDIENTS

- 1 ½ c. warm water
- 1 ¼ c. bread flour
- 2 tbsps. Honey
- 2 c. whole wheat flour
- 2 tsp. Yeast
- 1 ½ tbsps. Olive oil
- 1 tbsp. vinegar

NUTRITIONAL FACTS:

Calories: 228, Fat: 3.7 g, Carbs: 41.8 g, Protein: 6.9 g, Sugars: 0 g, Sodium: 15 mg

COOKING: 40'

PREPARATION: 5'

SERVES: 8

DIRECTIONS

1. In a bread machine, combine all ingredients, and then process on dough cycle. Once done, create 8 pieces shaped like a flattened ball. Create a donut shape using your thumb to make a hole at the center of each ball.

2. Place donut-shaped dough on a greased baking sheet then covers and let it rise about ½ hour. Prepare about 2 inches of water to boil in a large pan.

3. In boiling water, drop one at a time the bagels and boil for 1 minute, then turn them once. Remove them and return to the baking sheet and bake at 350oF for about 20 to 25 minutes until golden brown.

22. CEREAL WITH CRANBERRY-ORANGE TWIST

INGREDIENTS

- ½ c. water
- ½ c. orange juice
- 1/3 c. oat bran
- ¼ c. dried cranberries
- sugar as desired
- ½ cup milk

NUTRITIONAL FACTS:

Calories: 220, Fat: 2.4 g, Carbs: 43.5 g, Protein: 6.2 g, Sugars: 8 g, Sodium: 1 mg

COOKING: 0'

PREPARATION: 5'

SERVES: 1

DIRECTIONS

1. In a bowl, combine all ingredients. Put the bowl in the microwave for about 2 minutes, then serve with sugar and milk. Enjoy!

23. NO COOK OVERNIGHT OATS

INGREDIENTS

- 1 ½ c. low-fat milk
- 5 whole almond pieces
- 1 tsp. chia seeds
- 2 tbsps. Oats
- 1 tsp. sunflower seeds
- 1 tbsp. Craisins

NUTRITIONAL FACTS:

Calories: 271, Fat: 9.8 g, Carbs: 35.4 g, Protein: 16.7 g, Sugars: 9 g, Sodium: 103 mg

COOKING: 0'

PREPARATION: 5'

SERVES: 1

DIRECTIONS

1. In a jar or mason bottle with a cap, mix all ingredients. Refrigerate overnight. Enjoy for breakfast.

24. SIMPLE CHEESE AND BROCCOLI OMELETS

INGREDIENTS

- 3 tablespoons extra-virgin olive oil, divided
- 2 cups chopped broccoli
- 8 large eggs
- ¼ cup 1% milk
- ½ teaspoon freshly ground black pepper
- 8 tablespoons shredded reduced-fat Monterey Jack cheese, divided

NUTRITIONAL FACTS:

Calories: 292, Fat: 23 g, Carbs: 4 g, Fiber: 1 g, Protein: 18 g, Potassium: 308 mg, Sodium: 282 mg

COOKING: 10'

PREPARATION: 15'

SERVES: 4

DIRECTIONS

1. In a nonstick skillet, heat 1 tablespoon of oil over medium-high heat. Add the broccoli and sauté, occasionally stirring, for 3 to 5 minutes, or until the broccoli turns bright green. Scrape into a bowl.

2. Mix the eggs, milk, plus pepper in a small bowl. Wipe out the skillet and heat ½ tablespoon of oil. Add one-quarter of the egg mixture and tilt the skillet to ensure an even layer. Cook for 2 minutes and then add 2 tablespoons of cheese and one-quarter of the broccoli. Use a spatula to fold into an omelet.

3. Repeat step 3 with the remaining 1½ tablespoons of oil, remaining egg mixture, 6 tablespoons of cheese, and remaining broccoli to make a total of 4 omelets. Divide into 4 storage containers.

25. CREAMY AVOCADO AND EGG SALAD SANDWICHES

INGREDIENTS

- 2 small avocados, halved and pitted
- 2 tablespoons nonfat plain Greek yogurt
- Juice of 1 large lemon
- ¼ teaspoon salt
- ½ teaspoon freshly ground black pepper
- 8 large eggs, hardboiled, peeled, and chopped
- 3 tablespoons finely chopped fresh dill
- 3 tablespoons finely chopped fresh parsley
- 8 whole wheat bread slices (or your choice)

NUTRITIONAL FACTS:

Calories: 488, Fat: 22 g, Carbs: 48 g, Fiber: 8 g, Protein: 23 g, Sodium: 297 mg

COOKING: 15'

PREPARATION: 15'

SERVES: 4

DIRECTIONS

1. Scoop the avocados into a large bowl and mash. Mix in the yogurt, lemon juice, salt, and pepper. Add the eggs, dill, and parsley and combine.

2. Store the bread and salad separately in 4 reusable storage bags and 4 containers and assemble the night before or serving. To serve, divide the mixture evenly among 4 of the bread slices and top with the other slices to make sandwiches.

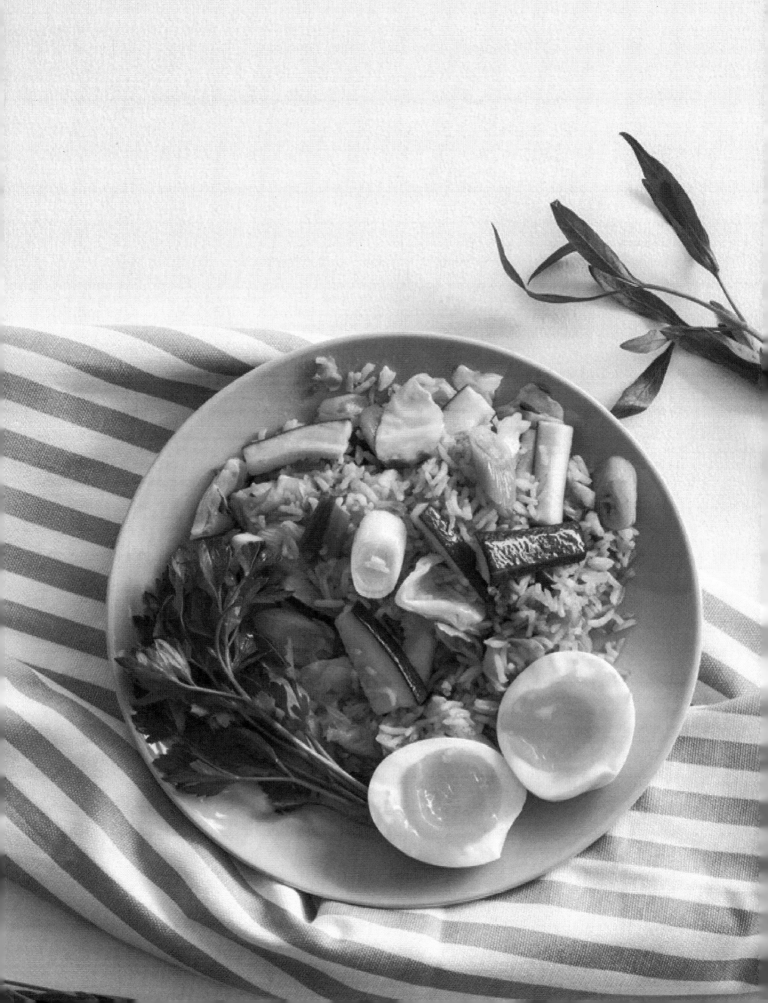

CHAPTER 11
LUNCH RECIPES

26. STUFFED EGGPLANT SHELLS

INGREDIENTS

- 1 medium eggplant
- 1 cup of water
- 1 tablespoon olive oil
- 4 oz. cooked white beans
- 1/4 cup onion, chopped
- 1/2 cup red, green, or yellow bell peppers, chopped
- 1 cup canned unsalted tomatoes
- 1/4 cup tomatoes liquid
- 1/4 cup celery, chopped
- 1 cup fresh mushrooms, sliced
- 3/4 cup whole-wheat breadcrumbs
- Freshly ground black pepper, to taste

NUTRITIONAL FACTS:

Calories: 334, Fat: 10 g, Sodium: 142 mg, Carbs: 35 g, Protein: 26 g

COOKING: 25'

PREPARATION: 10'

SERVES: 2

DIRECTIONS

1. Prepare the oven to 350 degrees F to preheat. Grease a baking dish with cooking spray and set it aside. Trim and cut the eggplant into half, lengthwise. Scoop out the pulp using a spoon and leave the shell about ¼ inch thick.

2. Place the shells in the baking dish with their cut side up. Add water to the bottom of the dish. Dice the eggplant pulp into cubes and set them aside. Add oil to an iron skillet and heat it over medium heat. Stir in onions, peppers, chopped eggplant, tomatoes, celery, mushrooms, and tomato juice.

3. Cook for 10 minutes on simmering heat, then stirs in beans, black pepper, and breadcrumbs. Divide this mixture into the eggplant shells. Cover the shells with a foil sheet and bake for 15 minutes. Serve warm.

27. SOUTHWESTERN VEGETABLES TACOS

INGREDIENTS

- 1 tablespoon olive oil
- 1 cup red onion, chopped
- 1 cup yellow summer squash, diced
- 1 cup green zucchini, diced
- 3 large garlic cloves, minced
- 4 medium tomatoes, seeded and chopped
- 1 jalapeno chili, seeded and chopped
- 1 cup fresh corn kernels
- 1 cup canned pinto, rinsed and drained
- 1/2 cup fresh cilantro, chopped
- 8 corn tortillas
- 1/2 cup smoke-flavored salsa

NUTRITIONAL FACTS:

Calories 310, Fat 6 g, Sodium 97 mg, Carbs 54 g, Protein 10 g

COOKING: 20'

PREPARATION: 10'

SERVES: 4

DIRECTIONS

1. Add olive oil to a saucepan, then heat it over medium heat. Stir in onion and sauté until soft. Add zucchini and summer squash. Cook for 5 minutes.

2. Stir in corn kernels, jalapeno, garlic, beans, and tomatoes. Cook for another 5 minutes. Stir in cilantro, then remove the pan from the heat.

3. Warm each tortilla in a dry nonstick skillet for 20 secs per side. Place the tortilla on the serving plate. Spoon the vegetable mixture in each tortilla. Top the mixture with salsa. Serve.

28. SEARED SCALLOPS WITH BLOOD ORANGE GLAZE

INGREDIENTS

- 3 tablespoons extra-virgin olive oil, divided
- 3 garlic cloves, minced
- ½ teaspoon kosher salt, divided
- 4 blood oranges, juiced
- 1 teaspoon blood orange zest
- ½ teaspoon red pepper flakes
- 1-pound scallops, small side muscle removed
- ¼ teaspoon freshly ground black pepper
- ¼ cup fresh chives, chopped

NUTRITIONAL FACTS:

Calories: 140, Fat: 4 g, Sodium: 570 mg, Carbohydrates: 12 g, Protein: 15 g

COOKING: 20'

PREPARATION: 15'

SERVES: 4

DIRECTIONS

1. Heat-up 1 tablespoon of the olive oil in a small saucepan over medium-high heat. Add the garlic and ¼ teaspoon of the salt and sauté for 30 seconds.

2. Add the orange juice and zest, bring to a boil, reduce the heat to medium-low, and cook within 20 minutes, or until the liquid reduces by half and becomes a thicker syrup consistency. Remove and mix in the red pepper flakes.

3. Pat the scallops dry with a paper towel and season with the remaining ¼ teaspoon salt and the black pepper. Heat-up the remaining 2 tablespoons of olive oil in a large skillet on medium-high heat. Add the scallops gently and sear.

4. Cook on each side within 2 minutes. If cooking in 2 batches, use 1 tablespoon of oil per batch. Serve the scallops with the blood orange glaze and garnish with the chives.

29. LEMON GARLIC SHRIMP

INGREDIENTS

- 2 tablespoons extra-virgin olive oil
- 3 garlic cloves, sliced
- ½ teaspoon kosher salt
- ¼ teaspoon red pepper flakes
- 1-pound large shrimp, peeled and deveined
- ½ cup white wine
- 3 tablespoons fresh parsley, minced
- Zest of ½ lemon
- Juice of ½ lemon

NUTRITIONAL FACTS:

Calories: 200, Fat: 9 g, Sodium: 310 mg, Carbohydrates: 3 g, Protein: 23 g

COOKING: 10'

PREPARATION: 15'

SERVES: 8

DIRECTIONS

1. Heat-up the olive oil in a wok or large skillet over medium-high heat. Add the garlic, salt, and red pepper flakes and sauté until the garlic starts to brown, 30 seconds to 1 minute.

2. Add the shrimp and cook within 2 to 3 minutes on each side. Pour in the wine and deglaze the wok, scraping up any flavorful brown bits, for 1 to 2 minutes. Turn off the heat; mix in the parsley, lemon zest, and lemon juice.

30. SHRIMP FRA DIAVOLO

INGREDIENTS

- 2 tablespoons extra-virgin olive oil
- 1 onion, diced small
- 1 fennel bulb, cored and diced small, plus ¼ cup fronds for garnish
- 1 bell pepper, diced small
- ½ teaspoon dried oregano
- ½ teaspoon dried thyme
- ½ teaspoon kosher salt
- ¼ teaspoon red pepper flakes
- 1 (14.5-ounce) can no-salt-added diced tomatoes
- 1-pound shrimp, peeled and deveined
- Juice of 1 lemon
- Zest of 1 lemon
- 2 tablespoons fresh parsley, chopped, for garnish

NUTRITIONAL FACTS:

Calories: 240, Fat: 9 g, Sodium: 335 mg, Carbohydrates: 13 g, Protein: 25 g

COOKING: 10'

PREPARATION: 15'

SERVES: 4

DIRECTIONS

1. Heat-up the olive oil in a large skillet or sauté pan over medium heat. Add the onion, fennel, bell pepper, oregano, thyme, salt, and red pepper flakes and sauté until translucent, about 5 minutes.

2. Drizzle the pan using the canned tomatoes' juice, scraping up any brown bits, and bringing to a boil. Add the diced tomatoes and the shrimp. Lower heat to a simmer within 3 minutes.

3. Turn off the heat. Add the lemon juice and lemon zest, and toss well to combine. Garnish with the parsley and the fennel fronds.

31. FISH AMANDINE

INGREDIENTS

- 4-ounce skinless tilapia, trout, or halibut fillets, 1/2- to 1-inch thick
- ¼ cup buttermilk
- ½ teaspoon dry mustard
- 1/8 teaspoon crushed red pepper
- 1 tablespoon butter, melted
- ¼ teaspoon salt
- ½ cup panko bread crumbs
- 2 tbsp chopped fresh parsley
- ¼ cup sliced almonds, coarsely chopped
- 2 tablespoons grated Parmesan cheese

NUTRITIONAL FACTS:

Calories: 209, Fat: 8.7 g, Sodium: 302 mg, Carbohydrates: 6.7 g, Protein: 26.2 g

COOKING: 15'

PREPARATION: 15'

SERVES: 4

DIRECTIONS

1. Defrost fish, if frozen. Preheat oven to 450oF. Grease a shallow baking pan; set aside. Rinse fish; pat dry with paper towels.

2. Pour buttermilk into a shallow dish. In an extra shallow dish, mix bread crumbs, dry mustard, parsley, and salt. Soak fish into buttermilk, then into crumb mixture, turning to coat. Put coated fish in the ready baking pan.

3. Flavor the fish with almonds plus Parmesan cheese; drizzle with melted butter. Sprinkle with crinkled red pepper. Bake for 5 minutes per 1/2-inch thickness of fish or until fish flakes easily when checked with a fork.

32. LEMON SALMON WITH KAFFIR LIME

INGREDIENTS

- A whole side of salmon fillet
- 1 thinly sliced lemon
- 2 kaffir torn lime leaves
- 1 quartered and bruised lemongrass stalk
- 1 ½ cups fresh coriander leaves

NUTRITIONAL FACTS:

Calories: 103, Protein: 18 g, Carbs: 43.5 g, Fat: 11.8 g, Sodium: 170 mg

COOKING: 30'

PREPARATION: 15'

SERVES: 8

DIRECTIONS

1. Warm-up oven to 350 F. Covers a baking pan with foil sheets, overlapping the sides (enough to fold over the fish).

2. Put the salmon on the foil, top with the lemon, lime leaves, the lemongrass, and 1 cup of the coriander leaves. Option: season with salt and pepper.

3. Bring the long side of the foil to the center before folding the seal. Roll the ends to close up the salmon. Bake for 30 minutes. Transfer the cooked fish to a platter. Top with fresh coriander. Serve with white or brown rice.

33. PORK ROAST AND CRANBERRY ROAST

INGREDIENTS

- 2 minced garlic cloves
- 1/2 tsp. grated ginger Black pepper
- 1/2 c. low-sodium veggie stock
- 1 1/2 lbs. pork loin roast
- 1 tbsp. coconut flour
- 1/2 c. cranberries
- Juice of 1/2 lemon

NUTRITIONAL FACTS:

Calories: 330, Fat: 13 g, Carbs: 13 g, Protein: 25 g, Sugars: 7 g, Sodium: 150 mg

COOKING: 30'

PREPARATION: 10'

SERVES: 4

DIRECTIONS

1. Put the stock in the little pan, get hot over medium-high heat, add black pepper, ginger, garlic, cranberries, fresh freshly squeezed lemon juice along using the flour, whisk well and cook for ten minutes.
2. Put the roast in the pan, add the cranberry sauce at the very top, introduce inside oven and bake at 375F for an hour and 20 minutes.
3. Slice the roast, divide it along using the sauce between plates and serve.
4. Enjoy!

34. EASY PORK CHOPS

INGREDIENTS

- 1 c. low-sodium chicken stock
- 1 tsp. sweet paprika
- 4 boneless pork chops
- 1/4 tsp. black pepper
- 1 tbsp. extra-virgin olive oil

NUTRITIONAL FACTS:

Calories: 272, Fat: 4 g, Carbs: 14 g, Protein: 17 g, Sugars: 0.2 g, Sodium: 68 mg

COOKING: 10'

PREPARATION: 10'

SERVES: 4

DIRECTIONS

1. Heat up a pan while using the oil over medium-high heat, add pork chops, brown them for 5 minutes on either sides, add paprika, black pepper and stock, toss, cook for fifteen minutes more, divide between plates and serve by using a side salad.

2. Enjoy!

35. GROUND BEEF WITH GREENS & TOMATOES

INGREDIENTS

- 1 tbsp. organic olive oil
- ½ of white onion, chopped
- 2 garlic cloves, chopped finely
- 1 jalapeño pepper, chopped finely
- 1 pound lean ground beef
- 1 teaspoon ground coriander
- 1 teaspoon ground cumin
- ½ teaspoon ground turmeric
- ½ teaspoon ground ginger
- ½ teaspoon ground cinnamon
- ½ teaspoon ground fennel seeds
- Salt and freshly ground black pepper, to taste
- 8 fresh cherry tomatoes, quartered
- 8 collard greens leaves, stemmed and chopped
- 1 teaspoon fresh lemon juice

NUTRITIONAL FACTS:

Calories: 150, Protein: 14 g, Fat: 6 g, Carbs: 4 g, Sodium: 135 mg

COOKING: 15'

PREPARATION: 15'

SERVES: 4

DIRECTIONS

1. Heat oil on medium heat using a big skillet.
2. Add onion and sauté for approximately 4 minutes.
3. Add garlic and jalapeño pepper and sauté for almost 1 minute.
4. Add beef and spices and cook for 6 minutes breaking into pieces while using spoon.
5. Stir in tomatoes and greens and cook, stirring gently for approximately 4 minutes.
6. Stir in lemon juice and take away from heat.

36. CURRIED BEEF MEATBALLS

INGREDIENTS

For Meatballs:

- 1 pound lean ground beef
- 2 organic eggs, bea10
- 3 tablespoons red onion, minced
- ¼ cup fresh basil leaves, chopped
- 1 (1-inch) fresh ginger piece, chopped finely
- 4 garlic cloves, chopped finely
- 3 Thai bird's eye chilies, minced
- 1 teaspoon coconut sugar
- 1 tablespoon red curry paste
- Salt, to taste
- 1 tablespoon fish sauce
- 2 tablespoons coconut oil

For Curry:

- 1 red onion, chopped
- Salt, to taste
- 4 garlic cloves, minced
- 1 (1-inch) fresh ginger piece, minced
- 2 Thai bird's eye chilies, minced
- 2 tablespoons red curry paste
- 1 (14-ounce) coconut milk
- Salt and freshly ground black pepper, to taste
- Lime wedges, for serving

NUTRITIONAL FACTS:

Calories: 185, Protein: 19 g, Fat: 6 g, Carbs: 8 g, Sodium: 23 mg

COOKING: 22'

PREPARATION: 20'

SERVES: 6

DIRECTIONS

1. For meatballs in a large bowl, add all ingredients except oil and mix till well combined.
2. Make small balls from mixture.
3. In a large skillet, melt coconut oil on medium heat.
4. Add meatballs and cook for approximately 3-5 minutes or till golden brown all sides.
5. Transfer the meatballs right into a bowl.
6. In the same skillet, add onion as well as a pinch of salt and sauté for around 5 minutes.
7. Add garlic, ginger and chilies and sauté for about 1 minute.
8. Add curry paste and sauté for almost 1 minute.
9. Add coconut milk and meatballs and convey to some gentle simmer.
10. Reduce the warmth to low and simmer, covered for approximately 10 minutes.
11. Serve using the topping of lime wedges.

37. CHICKEN THIGHS AND APPLES MIX

INGREDIENTS

- 3 cored and sliced apples
- 1 tbsp apple cider vinegar treatment
- ¾ c. natural apple juice
- ¼ tsp. pepper and salt
- 1 tbsp. grated ginger
- 8 chicken thighs
- 3 tbsps. Chopped onion

NUTRITIONAL FACTS:

Calories: 214, Fat: 3 g, Carbs: 14 g, Protein: 15 g, Sodium: 405 mg

COOKING: 60'

PREPARATION: 15'

SERVES: 4

DIRECTIONS

1. In a bowl, mix chicken with salt, pepper, vinegar, onion, ginger, and apple juice, toss well, cover, keep within the fridge for ten minutes, transfer with a baking dish, and include apples. Introduce inside the oven at 400 0F for just 1 hour. Divide between plates and serve. Enjoy!

38. THAI CHICKEN THIGHS

INGREDIENTS

- ½ c. Thai chili sauce
- 1 chopped green onions bunch
- 4 lbs. chicken thighs

NUTRITIONAL FACTS:

Calories: 220, Fat: 4 g, Carbs: 12 g, Protein: 10 g, Sodium: 870 mg

COOKING: 1H 5'

PREPARATION: 15'

SERVES: 6

DIRECTIONS

1. Heat a pan over medium-high heat. Add chicken thighs, brown them for 5 minutes on both sides Transfer to some baking dish, then add chili sauce and green onions and toss.

2. Introduce within the oven and bake at 4000F for 60 minutes. Divide everything between plates and serve. Enjoy!

39. FALLING "OFF" THE BONE CHICKEN

INGREDIENTS

- 6 peeled garlic cloves
- 1 tbsp. organic extra virgin coconut oil
- 2 tbsps. Lemon juice
- 1 ½ c. pacific organic bone chicken broth
- ¼ tsp freshly ground black pepper
- ½ tsp. sea flavored vinegar
- 1 whole organic chicken piece
- 1 tsp. paprika
- 1 tsp. dried thyme

NUTRITIONAL FACTS:

Calories: 664, Fat: 44 g, Carbs: 44 g, Protein: 27 g, Sugars: 0.1 g, Sodium: 800 mg

COOKING: 40'

PREPARATION: 15'

SERVES: 4

DIRECTIONS

1. Take a small bowl and toss in the thyme, paprika, pepper, and flavored vinegar and mix them. Use the mixture to season the chicken properly. Pour down the oil in your instant pot and heat it to shimmering; toss in the chicken with breast downward and let it cook for about 6-7 minutes

2. After the 7 minutes, flip over the chicken pour down the broth, garlic cloves, and lemon juice. Cook within 25 minutes on a high setting. Remove the dish from the cooker and let it stand for about 5 minutes before serving.

40. GARLIC PORK SHOULDER

INGREDIENTS

- 2 tsps. Sweet paprika
- 4 lbs. pork shoulder
- 3 tbsps. Extra virgin essential olive oil
- Black pepper
- 3 tbsps. Minced garlic

NUTRITIONAL FACTS:

Calories: 321, Fat: 6 g, Carbs: 12 g, Protein: 18 g, Sugars: 0 g, Sodium: 470 mg

COOKING: 4H

PREPARATION: 10'

SERVES: 6

DIRECTIONS

1. In a bowl, mix extra virgin extra virgin olive oil with paprika, black pepper and oil and whisk well.
2. Brush pork shoulder with this mix, arrange inside a baking dish and introduce inside oven at 425 0F for twenty or so minutes.
3. Reduce heat to 325 0F F and bake for 4 hours.
4. Slice the meat, divide it between plates and serve having a side salad.
5. Enjoy!

41. GRILLED FLANK STEAK WITH LIME VINAIGRETTE

INGREDIENTS

- 2 tablespoons lime juice, freshly squeezed
- 2 tablespoons extra virgin olive oil
- ½ teaspoon ground black pepper
- ¼ cup chopped fresh cilantro
- 1 tablespoon ground cumin
- ¼ teaspoon red pepper flakes
- ¾ pound flank steak

NUTRITIONAL FACTS:

Calories per Servings: 103, Protein: 13 g, **Car**bs: 1 g, Fat: 5 g, Saturated Fat: 1 g, Sodium: 73 mg

COOKING: 10'

PREPARATION: 10'

SERVES: 6

DIRECTIONS

1. Heat the grill to low medium heat
2. In a food processor, place all ingredients except for the cumin, red pepper flakes, and flank steak. Pulse until smooth. This will be the vinaigrette sauce. Set aside.
3. Season the flank steak with ground cumin and red pepper flakes and allow to marinate for at least 10 minutes.
4. Place the steak on the grill rack and cook for 5 minutes on each side. Cut into the center to check the doneness of the meat. You can also insert a meat thermometer to check the internal temperature.
5. Remove from the grill and allow to stand for 5 minutes.
6. Slice the steak to 2 inches long and toss the vinaigrette to flavor the meat.
7. Serve with salad if desired.

42. ASIAN PORK TENDERLOIN

INGREDIENTS

- 2 tablespoons sesame seeds
- 1 teaspoon ground coriander
- 1/8 teaspoon cayenne pepper
- 1/8 teaspoon celery seed
- ½ teaspoon minced onion
- ¼ teaspoon ground cumin
- 1/8 teaspoon ground cinnamon
- 1 tablespoon sesame oil
- 1-pound pork tenderloin sliced into 4 equal portions

NUTRITIONAL FACTS:

Calories: 248, Protein: 26 g, Carbs: 0 g, Fat: 16 g, Saturated Fat: 5 g, Sodium: 57 mg

COOKING: 15'

PREPARATION: 10'

SERVES: 4

DIRECTIONS

1. Preheat the oven to 4000F.

2. In a skillet, toast the sesame seeds over low heat and set aside. Allow the sesame seeds to cool.

3. In a bowl, combine the rest of the ingredients expect for the pork tenderloin. Stir in the toasted sesame seeds.

4. Place the pork tenderloin in a baking dish and rub the spices on both sides.

5. Place the baking dish with the pork in the oven and bake for 15 minutes or until the internal temperature of the meat reaches to 1700F.

6. Serve warm.

43. SIMPLE BEEF BRISKET AND TOMATO SOUP

INGREDIENTS

- 1 tablespoon olive oil
- 2 ½ pounds beef brisket, trimmed of fat and cut into 8 equal parts
- A dash of ground black pepper
- 1 ½ cups chopped onions
- 4 cloves of garlic, smashed
- 1 teaspoon dried thyme
- 1 cup ripe roma tomatoes, chopped
- ¼ cup red wine vinegar
- 1 cup beef stock, low sodium or home made

NUTRITIONAL FACTS:

Calories: 229, Protein: 31 g, Carbs: 6 g, Fat: 9 g, Saturated Fat: 3 g, Sodium: 184 mg

COOKING: 3H

PREPARATION: 10'

SERVES: 8

DIRECTIONS

1. In a heavy pot, heat the oil over medium-high heat.
2. Season the brisket with ground black pepper and place in the pot.
3. Cook while stirring constantly until the beef turns brown on all sides.
4. Stir in the onions and cook until fragrant. Add in the garlic and thyme and cook for another minute until fragrant.
5. Pour in the rest of the ingredients and bring to a boil.
6. Cook until the beef is tender. This may take about 3 hours or more.

44. RUSTIC BEEF AND BARLEY SOUP

INGREDIENTS

- 1 teaspoon olive oil
- 1-pound beef round steak, sliced into strips
- 2 cups yellow onion, chopped
- 1 cup diced celery
- 4 cloves of garlic, chopped
- 1 cup diced roma tomatoes
- ½ cup diced sweet potato
- ½ cup diced mushrooms
- 1 cup diced carrots
- ¼ cup uncooked barley
- 3 cups low sodium vegetable stock
- 1 teaspoon dried sage
- 1 paprika
- A dash of black pepper to taste
- 1 cup chopped kale

NUTRITIONAL FACTS:

Calories per Servings: 246, Protein: 21 g
Carbs: 24 g, Fat: 4 g, Saturated Fat: 1 g, Sodium: 13 mg

COOKING: 40'

PREPARATION: 10'

SERVES: 6

DIRECTIONS

1. In a large pot, heat the oil over medium flame and stir in the beef. Cook for 5 minutes while stirring constantly until all sides turn brown.
2. Stir in the onion, celery, and garlic until fragrant.
3. Add in the rest of the ingredients except for the kale.
4. Bring to a boil and cook for 30 minutes until everything is tender.
5. Stir in the kale last and cook for another 5 minutes

45. SOUTHWESTERN BEAN SALAD WITH CREAMY AVOCADO DRESSING

INGREDIENTS

- 1 head romaine lettuce, chopped
- 1 can no-salt-added black beans, drained
- 2 cups fresh corn kernels
- 2 cups grape tomatoes, halved
- 2 small avocados, halved and pitted 1 cup chopped fresh cilantro
- 1 cup nonfat plain Greek yogurt 8 scallions, chopped
- 3 garlic cloves, quartered zest, and juice of 1 large lime
- ½ teaspoon sugar

NUTRITIONAL FACTS:

Calories: 349 g, Fat: 11 g, Carbs: 53 g, Fiber: 16 g, Protein: 19 g, Sodium: 77 mg

COOKING: 0'

PREPARATION: 15'

SERVES: 4

DIRECTIONS

1. Mix the lettuce, beans, corn, and tomatoes in a large bowl. Toss you well combined. Divide the salad into 4 large storage containers. Put the avocado flesh into your blender or food processor.

2. Add the yogurt, scallions, garlic, lime zest and juice, and sugar. Blend until well combined. Divide the dressing into 4 condiment cups. To serve, toss the salad and the dressing.

46. COBB PASTA SALAD

INGREDIENTS

- 1-pound whole wheat rotini pasta
- 2 cups cooked chicken breast, chopped
- 8 low-sodium turkey bacon slices, cooked and chopped 4 scallions, sliced
- 1½ cups cherry tomatoes halved
- ¼ teaspoon freshly ground black pepper
- 4 hard-boiled eggs, peeled and coarsely chopped
- 1/3 cup crumbled blue cheese
- 1 cup frozen avocado cubes
- ¾ cup Greek Yogurt Dill Dressing

NUTRITIONAL FACTS:

Calories: 550 g, Fat: 18 g, Carbs: 62 g, Fiber: 9.5 g, Protein: 40 g, Sodium: 619 mg

COOKING: 10'

PREPARATION: 15'

SERVES: 6

DIRECTIONS

1. Cook the pasta until al dente as stated to package directions. Rinse under cold water, then drain. Mix the pasta, chicken, bacon, scallions, tomatoes, pepper in a large bowl. Toss until well combined.

2. Add the eggs and blue cheese and fold until mixed well. Divide the salad into 6 storage containers. Divide the avocado into 6 small storage containers. Make the dressing as directed and store in 6 condiment cups.

3. The night before you're planning on having a salad, add the portion off the avocado to the salad so they will be soft by mealtime the next day. Serve drizzled with the dressing.

47. EDAMAME SALAD WITH CORN AND CRANBERRIES

INGREDIENTS

- 1 1/4 cups shelled edamame
- 3/4 cup corn kernels
- 1 red or orange bell pepper, chopped
- 1/4 cup dried cranberries
- 1 shallot, finely diced
- 2 tablespoons red wine vinegar
- 1 tablespoon olive oil
- 1 teaspoon agave nectar
- 1 teaspoon no-salt-added prepared mustard
- Freshly ground black pepper, to taste

NUTRITIONAL FACTS:

Calories: 149, Fat: 5 g, Protein: 5 g, Sodium: 5 mg, Fiber: 3 g, Carbs: 22 g, Sugar: 10 g

COOKING: 0'

PREPARATION: 15'

SERVES: 4

DIRECTIONS

1. Place the edamame, corn, bell pepper, cranberries, and shallot in a mixing bowl and stir to combine. Mix the vinegar, oil, agave nectar, and mustard into a small mixing bowl.

2. Pour the dressing over the salad. Flavor with freshly ground black pepper, to taste. Serve.

48. WARM ASIAN SLAW

INGREDIENTS

- 1 tablespoon sesame oil
- 1 tablespoon peanut oil
- 2 sliced scallions
- 2 cloves garlic, minced
- 1 tablespoon minced fresh ginger
- 1 medium bok choy, chopped
- 2 medium carrots, shredded
- 1 tablespoon unflavored rice vinegar
- 1/2 teaspoon sugar
- 1/2 teaspoon ground white pepper
- 1/2 tablespoon toasted sesame seeds (optional)

NUTRITIONAL FACTS:

Calories: 112, Fat: 7 g, Protein: 3 g, Sodium: 72 mg, Fiber: 3 g, Carbs: 9 g, Sugar: 4 g

COOKING: 3'

PREPARATION: 15'

SERVES: 4

DIRECTIONS

1. Heat both oils in a skillet over medium. Add scallions, garlic, and ginger and cook, stirring, for 1 minute. Add bok choy and carrots and sauté for 2 minutes. Remove from heat.
2. Place contents in a bowl. Stir in vinegar, sugar, and pepper. Garnish with sesame seeds, if desired. Serve immediately.

49. TANGY THREE-BEAN SALAD WITH BARLEY

INGREDIENTS

- 1 cup uncooked pearled barley
- 21/4 cups water
- 2 cups of green beans, slice into 2-inch pieces
- 1 (15-ounce) can no-salt-added kidney beans
- 1 (15-ounce) can no-salt-added garbanzo beans
- 1 medium red bell pepper, diced
- 1 small onion, finely chopped
- 2 tablespoons chopped fresh cilantro or parsley
- 1/3 cup canola oil
- 1/3 cup apple cider vinegar
- 1/3 cup pure maple syrup
- Freshly ground black pepper, to taste

NUTRITIONAL FACTS:

Calories: 367, Fat: 11 g, Protein: 11 g, Sodium: 10 mg, Fiber: 11 g, Carbs: 57 g, Sugar: 11 g

COOKING: 30'

PREPARATION: 15'

SERVES: 8

DIRECTIONS

1. Measure the barley and water into a saucepan and boil over high heat. Once boiling, adjust heat to low, cover, and simmer until water is absorbed, 25–30 minutes. Remove pan from heat, then drain and rinse well.

2. Put the green beans in a bowl, then put the drained canned beans, bell pepper, onion, barley, and chopped cilantro or parsley. Stir well.

3. Mix the oil, vinegar, plus maple syrup in a small mixing bowl. Put on the salad and toss to coat. Flavor with ground black pepper, then serve.

50. TUNA SALAD-STUFFED TOMATOES WITH ARUGULA

INGREDIENTS

- 1 teaspoon dried thyme
- 3 tablespoons sherry vinegar
- 3 tablespoons extra-virgin olive oil
- 1/3 cup chopped celery
- ¼ teaspoon freshly ground pepper
- 4 large tomatoes
- 8 cups baby arugula
- ¼ cup finely chopped red onion
- ¼ teaspoon salt
- ¼ cup chopped Kalamata olives
- 2 5-oz cans chunk light tuna in olive oil, drained
- 1 can great northern beans, rinsed

NUTRITIONAL FACTS:

Calories: 353, Fat: 17.6 g, Sodium: 501 mg, Carbs: 29.9 g, Protein: 19.7 g

COOKING: 15'

PREPARATION: 5'

SERVES: 4

DIRECTIONS

1. Whisk oil, salt, vinegar, and pepper in an average-sized bowl. Put 3 tablespoons of the dressing in a big bowl and set aside.

2. Slice enough off the top of each tomato to remove the core, chop enough of the tops to equal ½ cup and add to the average-sized bowl. Scoop out the soft tomato tissue using a teaspoon or melon baller and discard the pulp

3. Add tuna, onion, thyme, olives, and celery to the average-sized bowl; gently toss to mix. Fill the scooped tomatoes with the tuna mixture. Add beans and arugula to the gauze in the large bowl and toss to combine. Divide the salad into four plates and top each with a stuffed tomato.

51. STEAMED VEGGIE AND LEMON PEPPER SALMON

INGREDIENTS

- 1 carrot, peeled and julienned
- 1 red bell pepper, julienned
- 1 zucchini, julienned
- ½ lemon, sliced thinly
- 1 tsp pepper
- ½ tsp salt
- 1/2-lb salmon filet with skin on
- A dash of tarragon

NUTRITIONAL FACTS:

Calories: 216.2, Carbs: 4.1 g, Protein: 35.1 g, Fats: 6.6 g, Sodium: 332 mg

COOKING: 15'

PREPARATION: 15'

SERVES: 4

DIRECTIONS

1. In a heat-proof dish that fits inside a saucepan, add salmon with skin side down. Season with pepper. Add slices of lemon on top.

2. Place the julienned vegetables on top of salmon and season with tarragon. Cover top of fish with remaining cherry tomatoes and place dish on the trivet. Cover dish with foil. Cover pan and steam for 15 minutes. Serve and enjoy.

52. STEAMED FISH WITH SCALLIONS AND GINGER

INGREDIENTS

- ¼ cup chopped cilantro
- ¼ cup julienned scallions
- 2 tbsp julienned ginger
- 1 tbsp peanut oil
- 1-lb Tilapia filets
- 1 tsp garlic
- 1 tsp minced ginger
- 2 tbsp rice wine
- 1 tbsp low sodium soy sauce

NUTRITIONAL FACTS:

Calories: 219, Carbs: 4.5 g, Protein: 31.8 g, Fats: 8.2 g, Sodium: 252 mg

COOKING: 15'

PREPARATION: 15'

SERVES: 3

DIRECTIONS

1. Mix garlic, minced ginger, rice wine, and soy sauce in a heat-proof dish that fits inside a saucepan. Add the Tilapia filet and marinate for half an hour while turning over at the half time.

2. Cover dish of fish with foil and place on a trivet. Cover pan and steam for 15 minutes. Serve and enjoy.

53. STEAMED TILAPIA WITH GREEN CHUTNEY

INGREDIENTS

- 1-pound tilapia fillets, divided into 3
- ½ cup green commercial chutney

NUTRITIONAL FACTS:

Calories: 151.5, Carbs: 1.1 g, Protein: 30.7 g, Fats: 2.7 g, Sodium: 79 mg

COOKING: 10'

PREPARATION: 15'

SERVES: 3

DIRECTIONS

1. Cut 3 pieces of 15-inch lengths foil. In one foil, place one filet in the middle and 1/3 of chutney. Fold over the foil and seal the filet inside. Repeat process for remaining fish. Put packet on the trivet. Steam for 10 minutes. Serve and enjoy.

54. CREAMY HADDOCK WITH KALE

INGREDIENTS

- 1 tbsp olive oil
- 1 onion, chopped
- 2 cloves of garlic, minced
- 2 cups chicken broth
- 1 teaspoon crushed red pepper flakes
- 1-pound wild Haddock fillets
- ½ cup heavy cream
- 1 tablespoon basil
- 1 cup kale leaves, chopped
- Pepper to taste

NUTRITIONAL FACTS:

Calories: 130.5, Carbs: 5.5 g, Protein: 35.7 g, Fats: 14.5 g, Sodium: 278 mg

COOKING: 10'

PREPARATION: 15'

SERVES: 5

DIRECTIONS

1. Place a pot on medium-high fire within 3 minutes. Put oil, then sauté the onion and garlic for 5 minutes. Put the rest of the fixing, except for basil, and mix well. Boil on lower fire within 5 minutes. Serve with a sprinkle of basil.

55. STEWED COD FILET WITH TOMATOES

INGREDIENTS

- 1 tbsp olive oil
- 1 onion, sliced
- 1 ½ pound fresh cod fillets
- Pepper
- 1 lemon juice, freshly squeezed
- 1 can diced tomatoes

NUTRITIONAL FACTS:

Calories: 106.4, Carbs: 2.5 g, Protein: 17.8 g, Fats: 2.8 g, Sodium: 381 mg

COOKING: 15'

PREPARATION: 15'

SERVES: 6

DIRECTIONS

1. Sauté the onion for 2 minutes in a pot on medium-high fire. Stir in diced tomatoes and cook for 5 minutes. Add cod filet and season with pepper. Simmer on lower fire within 5 minutes. Serve with freshly squeezed lemon juice.

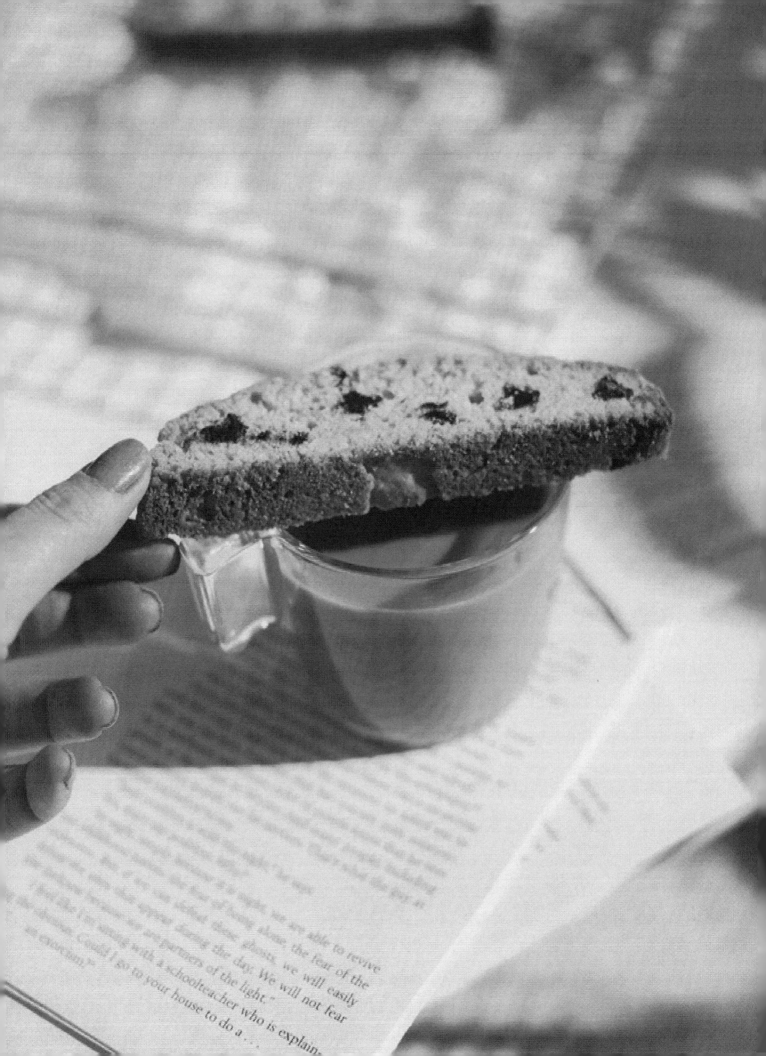

CHAPTER 12
SNACK RECIPES

56. MINI TERIYAKI TURKEY SANDWICHES

INGREDIENTS

- 2 chicken breast halves
- 1 cup soy sauce, low-salt
- ¼ cup cider vinegar
- 3 minced garlic cloves
- 1 tablespoon fresh ginger root
- 2 tablespoons cornstarch
- 20 Hawaiian sweet rolls
- ½ teaspoon pepper
- 2 tablespoons melted butter

NUTRITIONAL FACTS:

Calories: 252, Fat: 5 g, Carbs: 25 g, Net Carbs: 24 g, Protein: 26 g, Fiber: 1g, Sodium: 42 mg

COOKING: 30'

PREPARATION: 20'

SERVES: 20

DIRECTIONS

1. Put turkey in pressure cooker and combine the first six ingredients over it.
2. Cook it on manual for 25 minutes, and when finished, natural pressure release.
3. Push sauté after removing the turkey, then mix cornstarch and water, stirring into cooking juices, and cook until sauce is thickened. Shred meat and stir to heat.
4. You can split the rolls, buttering each side, and bake till golden brown, adding the meat mixture to the top.

57. PEACH CRUMBLE MUFFINS

INGREDIENTS

For the crumble:
- 2 tablespoons dark brown sugar
- 1 tablespoon honey
- 1 teaspoon ground cinnamon
- 2 tablespoons canola oil
- ½ cup old-fashioned rolled oats

For the peach muffins:
- 1 teaspoon baking powder
- 1 teaspoon baking soda
- 1 teaspoon ground cinnamon
- ½ teaspoon ground ginger
- ½ teaspoon kosher or sea salt
- ¼ cup canola oil
- ¼ cup dark brown sugar
- 2 large eggs
- 1½ teaspoons vanilla extract
- ¼ cup plain nonfat Greek yogurt
- 3 peaches, diced (about 1½ cups)
- 1¾ cups whole-wheat flour or whole-wheat pastry flour

NUTRITIONAL FACTS:

Calories: 187, Fat: 8 g, Sodium: 216 mg, Carbs: 26 g, Fiber: 3 g, Sugar: 10 g, Protein: 4 g

COOKING: 25'

PREPARATION: 25'

SERVES: 12

DIRECTIONS

1. In a small bowl, mix the brown sugar, honey, cinnamon, canola oil, and oats until combined for the crumble. For your muffins, mix the flour, baking powder, baking soda, cinnamon, ginger, and salt in a large bowl.

2. Beat the canola oil, brown sugar, and one egg at a time in a separate bowl, using a hand mixer until fluffy. Beat in the vanilla extract and yogurt. Put the flour mixture in the bowl and whisk until the ingredients are just combined.

3. Fold in the diced peaches with a spatula. Preheat the oven to 425°F. Oiled a 12-cup muffin tin with muffin liners. Fill each muffin well with batter about three-quarters of the way full. Scoop the crumble batter on top of each.

4. Bake for 5 to 6 minutes, then reduce the oven temperature to 350°F and bake for 15 to 18 additional minutes. Cool before removing from the muffin tin. Once completely cooled, serve.

58. PEANUT BUTTER BANANA BREAD BITES

INGREDIENTS

- 1½ cups whole-wheat pastry flour
- 2 tablespoons ground flaxseed
- 1 teaspoon baking powder
- ½ teaspoon kosher or sea salt
- ½ teaspoon ground cinnamon
- 3 ripe bananas, peeled
- 2 large eggs
- 2 tablespoons canola oil
- ½ cup dark brown sugar
- 2 tablespoons honey
- ½ cup natural creamy peanut butter
- ¼ cup nonfat Greek yogurt
- 1 teaspoon vanilla extract
- ¼ cup unsalted roasted peanuts, crushed

NUTRITIONAL FACTS:

Calories: 123, Fat: 5 g, Sodium: 81 mg, Carbs: 17 g, Fiber: 2 g, Sugar: 8 g, Protein: 3 g

COOKING: 20'

PREPARATION: 10'

SERVES: 24

DIRECTIONS

1. Preheat the oven to 350°F. Oiled a 24-cup mini muffin tin with cooking spray. In a bowl, whisk the flour, flaxseed, baking powder, salt, and cinnamon. Beat the bananas in a separate bowl with a hand mixer set on low.

2. Add the eggs, one at a time, then add the canola oil, brown sugar, and honey. Adjust the speed to medium and beat until fluffy. Add the peanut butter, Greek yogurt, and vanilla extract and mix until combined. Lower the speed to low, then beat in the dry ingredient mixture until just combined.

3. Put the mixture into each of the muffin wells about three-quarters of the way full. Tap it on the counter until the batter is evenly spread out.

4. Top with the crushed peanuts. Bake within 20 minutes, until a toothpick inserted into the center of a bite, comes out clean. Let rest on the counter until cooled. Remove the bites from the muffin tin. Serve.

59. TOASTED ALMOND AMBROSIA

INGREDIENTS

- ½ Cup Almonds, Slivered
- ½ Cup Coconut, Shredded & Unsweetened
- 3 Cups Pineapple, Cubed
- 5 Oranges, Segment
- 2 Red Apples, Cored & Diced
- 2 Tablespoons Cream Sherry
- Mint Leaves, Fresh to Garnish
- 1 Banana, Halved Lengthwise, Peeled & Sliced

NUTRITIONAL FACTS:

Calories: 177, Fat: 4.9 g, Sodium: 13 mg, Carbs: 36 g, Fiber: 0 g, Sugar: 0 g, Protein: 3.4 g

COOKING: 20'

PREPARATION: 10'

SERVES: 2

DIRECTIONS

1. Start by heating your oven to 325, and then get out a baking sheet. Roast your almonds for ten minutes, making sure they're spread out evenly. Transfer them to a plate and then toast your coconut on the same baking sheet.

2. Toast for ten minutes. Mix your banana, sherry, oranges, apples, and pineapple in a bowl. Divide the mixture, not serving bowls and top with coconut and almonds. Garnish with mint before serving.

60. ZESTY ZUCCHINI MUFFINS

INGREDIENTS

- Vegetable oil cooking spray
- ½ cup of sugar
- ¼ teaspoon iodized salt
- ¼ teaspoon ground nutmeg
- ¾ cup skim milk
- 1 cup shredded zucchini
- 1 tablespoon baking powder
- 1 large egg
- 2 teaspoons grated lemon rind
- 2 cups of all-purpose flour
- 3 tablespoons vegetable oil

NUTRITIONAL FACTS:

Calories: 169, Sodium: 211.5 mg, Fats: 4.8 g, Potassium: 80.2 g, Carbs: 29.1 g, Fibers: 2.5 g, Sugar: 12.8 g, Proteins: 0 g

COOKING: 30'

PREPARATION: 15'

SERVES: 12

DIRECTIONS

1. Mix the flour, baking powder, sugar, salt, plus lemon rinds in a bowl. Create a well in the center of the flour batter. In another bowl, mix zucchini, milk, vegetable oil, and egg. Coat muffin cups with vegetable oil cooking spray.

2. Divide the batter equally into 12 muffin cups. Transfer the muffin cups to the baking pan, put it in a microwave oven, and bake at 400 °F within 30 minutes until light golden brown. Remove, then allow to cool on a wire rack before serving.

61. BLUEBERRY OAT MUFFINS

INGREDIENTS

For the crumble:

- ½ cup raw oatmeal
- ½ teaspoon baking powder
- ½ teaspoon iodized salt
- ½ cup dry milk
- ¼ cup of vegetable oil
- ¼ teaspoon baking soda
- 1/3 cup sugar
- 1 ½ cup flour
- 1 cup milk
- 1 cup blueberries

NUTRITIONAL FACTS:

Calories: 150, Sodium: 180 mg, Fats: 5 g, Carbohydrates: 22 g, Proteins: 4 g, Fibers: 1 g

COOKING: 30'

PREPARATION: 15'

SERVES: 12

DIRECTIONS

1. Preheat oven to 350 °F. Coat the muffin tins with vegetable oil. Mix or combine the flour, baking soda, baking powder, oats, sugar, and salt in a bowl. Mix milk, dry milk, egg, and vegetable oil in another bowl.

2. Pour the bowl of wet fixing into the bowl of dry fixing and mix partially. Add the blueberries and mix until the consistency turns lumpy. Scoop blueberry batter into the muffin tins.

3. Bake within 30 minutes until the muffins turn golden brown on the edges. Serve warm immediately or put it in an airtight container and store it in the refrigerator to chill.

62. BANANA BREAD

INGREDIENTS

- Vegetable oil cooking spray
- ½ cup brown rice flour
- ½ cup amaranth flour
- ½ cup tapioca flour
- ½ cup millet flour
- ½ cup quinoa flour
- ½ cup of raw sugar
- ¾ cup egg whites
- 1/8 teaspoon iodized salt
- 1 teaspoon baking soda
- 2 tablespoons grapeseed oil
- 2 pieces of mashed banana

NUTRITIONAL FACTS:

Calories: 150, Sodium: 150 mg, Fats: 3 g, Fibers: 2 g, Proteins: 4 g, Sugar: 7 g

COOKING: 60'

PREPARATION: 15'

SERVES: 14

DIRECTIONS

1. Preheat oven to 350 °F. Coat a loaf pan with a vegetable oil cooking spray, dust evenly with a bit of flour, and set aside. In a bowl, mix the brown rice flour, amaranth flour, tapioca flour, millet flour, quinoa flour, and baking soda.

2. Coat a separate bowl with vegetable oil, then mix eggs, sugar, and mashed bananas. Pour the bowl of wet fixing into the bowl of dry fixing and mix thoroughly. Scoop the mixture into the loaf pan. Bake within an hour.

3. To check the doneness, insert a toothpick in the center of the loaf pan; if you remove the toothpick and it has no batter sticking to it, remove the bread from the oven. Slice and serve immediately and store the remaining banana bread in a refrigerator to prolong shelf life.

63. MILK CHOCOLATE PUDDING

INGREDIENTS

- ½ teaspoon vanilla extract
- 1/3 cup chocolate chips
- 1/8 teaspoon salt
- 2 cups nonfat milk
- 2 tablespoons cocoa powder
- 2 tablespoons sugar
- 3 tablespoons cornstarch

NUTRITIONAL FACTS:

Calories: 197, Sodium: 5 mg, Fats: 5 g, Carbs: 9 g, Proteins: 0.5 g

COOKING: 15'

PREPARATION: 15'

SERVES: 4

DIRECTIONS

1. Mix cocoa powder, cornstarch, sugar, and salt in a saucepan and whisk in milk; frequently stir over medium heat.

2. Remove, put the chocolate chips and vanilla extract, stir until the chocolate chips and vanilla melt into the pudding. Pour contents into serving bowls and store in a chiller. Serve chilled.

64. MINTY LIME AND GRAPEFRUIT YOGURT PARFAIT

INGREDIENTS

- A handful of torn mint leaves
- 2 teaspoons grated lime zest
- 2 tablespoons lime juice extract
- 3 tablespoons raw honey
- 4 large red grapefruits
- 4 cups reduced-fat plain yogurt

NUTRITIONAL FACTS:

Calories: 207, Sodium: 115 mg, Fats: 3 g, Cholesterol: 10 mg, Carbs: 39 mg, Sugar: 36 g, Fibers: 3 g

COOKING: 0'

PREPARATION: 15'

SERVES: 6

DIRECTIONS

1. Cut the top and lower part of the red grapefruits and stand the fruit upright on a cutting board. Discard the peel with a knife and slice along the membrane of each segment to remove the skin.

2. Mix yogurt, lime juice extract, and lime zest in a bowl. Layer half of the grapefruit and yogurt mixture into 6 parfait glasses; add another layer until the glass is filled and then drizzle with honey and top with mint leaves. Serve immediately.

65. PEACH TARTS

INGREDIENTS

Tart Ingredients:

- ¼ cup softened butter
- ¼ teaspoon ground nutmeg
- 1 cup all-purpose flour
- 3 tablespoons sugar

Filling Ingredients:

- ¼ teaspoon ground cinnamon
- ¼ cup coarsely chopped almonds
- 1/8 teaspoon almond extract
- 1/3 cup sugar
- 2 pounds peaches medium, peeled, thinly sliced

NUTRITIONAL FACTS:

Calories: 222, Sodium: 46 mg, Fats: 8 g, Cholesterol: 15 mg, Carbs: 36 g, Sugar: 21 g, Fibers: 3 g, Proteins: 4 g

COOKING: 55'

PREPARATION: 15'

SERVES: 8

DIRECTIONS

1. Preheat oven to 375 °F. Mix butter, nutmeg, and sugar in a bowl until light and fluffy. Add and beat in flour until well-blended. Place the batter on an ungreased fluted tart baking pan and press firmly on the bottom and topsides.

2. Put it in the medium rack of the preheated oven and bake for about 10 minutes until it turns to a crust. In a bowl, coat peaches with sugar, flour, cinnamon, almond extract, and almonds.

3. Open the oven, put the tart crust on the lower rack of the oven, and pour in the peach filling; bake for about 40-45 minutes. Remove, cool, and serve; or cover with a cling wrap and refrigerate to serve chilled.

66. RASPBERRY NUTS PARFAIT

INGREDIENTS

- ¼ cup frozen raspberries
- ¼ cup frozen blueberries
- ¼ cup toasted, thinly sliced almonds
- 1 cup nonfat, plain Greek yogurt
- 2 teaspoons raw honey

NUTRITIONAL FACTS:

Calories: 378, Sodium: 83 mg, Fats: 15 g, Fibers: 6 g, Carbs: 35 g, Proteins: 30 g, Sugar: 25 g

COOKING: 10'

PREPARATION: 15'

SERVES: 1

DIRECTIONS

1. First, layer Greek yogurt in a parfait glass; add berries; layer yogurt again, top with almonds and more berries; drizzle with honey. Serve chilled.

67. APRICOT BISCOTTI

INGREDIENTS

- 2 Tablespoons Honey, Dark
- 2 Tablespoons Olive Oil
- ½ Teaspoon Almond Extract
- ¼ Cup Almonds, Chopped Roughly
- 2/3 Cup Apricots, Dried
- 2 Tablespoons Milk, 1% & Low Fat
- 2 Eggs, Beaten Lightly
- ¾ Cup Whole Wheat Flour
- ¾ Cup All-Purpose Flour
- ¼ Cup Brown Sugar, Packed Firm
- 1 Teaspoon Baking Powder

NUTRITIONAL FACTS:

Calories: 291, Fat: 2 g, Sodium: 123 mg, Carbs: 12 g, Fiber: 0 g, Sugar: 0 g, Protein: 2 g

COOKING: 50'

PREPARATION: 10'

SERVES: 4

DIRECTIONS

1. Start by heating the oven to 350, then mix your baking powder, brown sugar, and flours in a bowl. Whisk your canola oil, eggs, almond extract, honey, and milk. Mix until it forms a smooth dough. Fold in the apricots and almonds.

2. Put your dough on plastic wrap, and then roll it out to a twelve-inch-long and three-inch wide rectangle. Place this dough on a baking sheet, and bake for twenty-five minutes. It should turn golden brown. Allow it to cool, slice it into ½ inch thick slices, and then bake for another fifteen minutes. It should be crispy.

68. APPLE & BERRY COBBLER

INGREDIENTS

Filling:

- 1 Cup Blueberries, Fresh
- 2 Cups Apples, Chopped
- 1 Cup Raspberries, Fresh
- 2 Tablespoons Brown Sugar
- 1 Teaspoon Lemon Zest
- 2 Teaspoon Lemon Juice, Fresh
- ½ Teaspoon Ground Cinnamon
- 1 ½ Tablespoons Corn Starch

Topping:

- ¾ Cup Whole Wheat Pastry Flour
- 1 ½ Tablespoon Brown Sugar
- ½ Teaspoon Vanilla Extract, Pure
- ¼ Cup Soy Milk
- ¼ Teaspoon Sea Salt, Fine
- 1 Egg White

NUTRITIONAL FACTS:

Calories: 131, Fat: 0 g, Sodium: 14 mg, Carbs: 13.8 g, Fiber: 0 g, Sugar: 0 g, Protein: 7.2 g

COOKING: 40'

PREPARATION: 10'

SERVES: 4

DIRECTIONS

1. Turn your oven to 350, and get out six small ramekins. Grease them with cooking spray. Mix your lemon juice, lemon zest, blueberries, sugar, cinnamon, raspberries, and apples in a bowl. Stir in your cornstarch, mixing until it dissolves.

2. Beat your egg white in a different bowl, whisking it with sugar, vanilla, soy milk, and pastry flour. Divide your berry mixture between the ramekins and top with the vanilla topping. Put your ramekins on a baking sheet, baking for thirty minutes. The top should be golden brown before serving.

69. MIXED FRUIT COMPOTE CUPS

INGREDIENTS

- 1 ¼ Cup Water
- ½ Cup Orange juice
- 12 Ounces Mixed Dried Fruit
- 1 Teaspoon Ground Cinnamon
- ¼ Teaspoon Ground Ginger
- ¼ Teaspoon Ground Nutmeg
- 4 Cups Vanilla Frozen Yogurt, Fat-Free

NUTRITIONAL FACTS:

Calories: 228, Fat: 5.7 g, Cholesterol: 15 mg, Sodium: 114 mg, Carbs: 12.4 g, Fiber: 0 g, Sugar: 0 g, Protein: 9.1 g

COOKING: 15'

PREPARATION: 5'

SERVES: 2

DIRECTIONS

1. Mix your dried fruit, nutmeg, cinnamon, water, orange juice, and ginger in a saucepan. Cover, and allow it to cook over medium heat for ten minutes. Remove the cover and then cook for another ten minutes. Add your frozen yogurt to serving cups, and top with the fruit mixture.

70. GENEROUS GARLIC BREAD STICK

INGREDIENTS

- ¼ cup almond butter, softened
- 1 teaspoon garlic powder
- 2 cups almond flour
- ½ tablespoon baking powder
- 1 tablespoon Psyllium husk powder
- ¼ teaspoon sunflower seeds
- 3 tablespoons almond butter, melted
- 1 egg
- ¼ cup boiling water

NUTRITIONAL FACTS:

Total Carbs: 7 g, Fiber: 2 g, Protein: 7 g, Fat: 24 g, Sodium: 24 mg

COOKING: 15'

PREPARATION: 15'

SERVES: 8

DIRECTIONS

1. Pre-heat your oven to 400 degrees F.
2. Line baking sheet with parchment paper and keep it on the side.
3. Beat almond butter with garlic powder and keep it on the side.
4. Add almond flour, baking powder, husk, sunflower seeds in a bowl and mix in almond butter and egg, mix well.
5. Pour boiling water in the mix and stir until you have a nice dough.
6. Divide the dough into 8 balls and roll into breadsticks.
7. Place on baking sheet and bake for 15 minutes.
8. Brush each stick with garlic almond butter and bake for 5 minutes more.
9. Serve and enjoy!

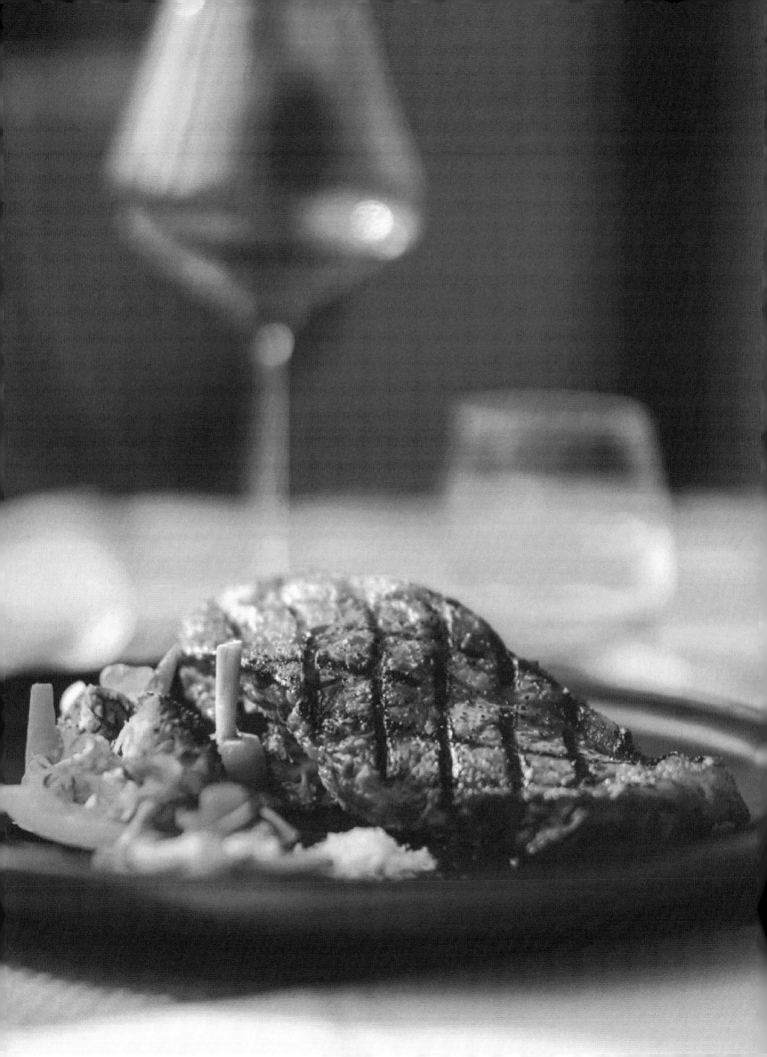

CHAPTER 13
DINNER RECIPES

71. SWEET-GINGER SCALLOPS

INGREDIENTS

- 1-pound sea scallops, shells removed
- ½ cup coconut aminos
- 3 tablespoons maple syrup
- ½ teaspoon garlic powder
- ½ teaspoon ground ginger

NUTRITIONAL FACTS:

Calories: 233.4, Carbs: 23.7 g
Protein: 31.5 g, Fats: 1.4 g, Sodium: 153 mg

COOKING: 15'

PREPARATION: 15'

SERVES: 3

DIRECTIONS

1. In a heat-proof dish that fits inside a saucepan, add all ingredients. Mix well. Cover dish of scallops with foil and place on a trivet. Cover pan and steam for 10 minutes. Let it stand in the pan for another 5 minutes. Serve and enjoy

72. SAVORY LOBSTER ROLL

INGREDIENTS

- 1 ½ cups chicken broth, low sodium
- 2 teaspoon old bay seasoning
- 2 pounds lobster tails, raw and in the shell
- 1 lemon, halved
- 3 scallions, chopped
- 1 teaspoon celery seeds

NUTRITIONAL FACTS:

Calories: 209, Carbs: 1.9 g, Protein: 38.2 g, Fats: 5.4 g, Sodium: 288 mg

COOKING: 20'

PREPARATION: 15'

SERVES: 6

DIRECTIONS

1. Place a heavy-bottomed pot on medium-high fire and add all ingredients and ½ of the lemon. Cover, bring to a boil, lower fire to a simmer, and simmer for 15 minutes. Let it rest for another 5 minutes. Serve and enjoy with freshly squeezed lemon juice.

73. GARLIC AND TOMATOES ON MUSSELS

INGREDIENTS

- ¼ cup white wine
- ½ cup of water
- 3 Roma tomatoes, chopped
- 2 cloves of garlic, minced
- 1 bay leaf
- 2 pounds mussels, scrubbed
- ½ cup fresh parsley, chopped
- 1 tbsp oil
- Pepper

NUTRITIONAL FACTS:

Calories: 172.8, Carbs: 10.2 g, Protein: 19.5 g, Fats: 6 g, Sodium: 261 mg

COOKING: 15'

PREPARATION: 15'

SERVES: 6

DIRECTIONS

1. Warm a pot on medium-high fire within 3 minutes. Put oil and stir around to coat pot with oil. Sauté the garlic, bay leaf, and tomatoes for 5 minutes.

2. Add remaining ingredients except for parsley and mussels. Mix well. Add mussels. Cover, and boil for 5 minutes. Serve with a sprinkle of parsley and discard any unopened mussels.

74. OVEN-FRIED CHICKEN BREASTS

INGREDIENTS

- ½ pack Ritz crackers
- 1 c. plain non-fat yogurt
- 8 boneless, skinless, and halved chicken breasts

NUTRITIONAL FACTS:

Calories: 200, Fat: 13 g, Carbs: 98 g, Protein: 19 g, Sodium: 217 mg

COOKING: 30'

PREPARATION: 15'

SERVES: 8

DIRECTIONS

1. Preheat the oven to 350 0F. Rinse and pat dry the chicken breasts. Pour the yogurt into a shallow bowl. Dip the chicken pieces in the yogurt, then roll in the cracker crumbs. Place the chicken in a single layer in a baking dish. Bake within 15 minutes per side. Serve.

75. ROSEMARY ROASTED CHICKEN

INGREDIENTS

- 8 rosemary springs
- 1 minced garlic clove
- Black pepper
- 1 tbsp. chopped rosemary
- 1 chicken
- 1 tbsp. organic olive oil

NUTRITIONAL FACTS:

Calories: 325, Fat: 5 g, Carbs: 15 g, Protein: 14 g, Sodium: 950 mg

COOKING: 20'

PREPARATION: 15'

SERVES: 8

DIRECTIONS

1. In a bowl, mix garlic with rosemary, rub the chicken with black pepper, the oil and rosemary mix, place it inside roasting pan, introduce inside the oven at 350 0F, and roast for sixty minutes and 20 min. Carve chicken, divide between plates and serve using a side dish. Enjoy!

76. ARTICHOKE AND SPINACH CHICKEN

INGREDIENTS

- 10 oz baby spinach
- ½ tsp. crushed red pepper flakes
- 14 oz. chopped artichoke hearts
- 28 oz. no-salt-added tomato sauce
- 2 tbsps. Essential olive oil
- 4 boneless and skinless chicken breasts

NUTRITIONAL FACTS:

Calories: 212, Fat: 3 g, Carbs: 16 g, Protein: 20 g, Sugars: 5 g, Sodium: 418 mg

COOKING: 5'

PREPARATION: 15'

SERVES: 4

DIRECTIONS

1. Heat-up a pan with the oil over medium-high heat, add chicken and red pepper flakes and cook for 5 minutes on them. Add spinach, artichokes, and tomato sauce, toss, cook for ten minutes more, divide between plates and serve. Enjoy!

77. PUMPKIN AND BLACK BEANS CHICKEN

INGREDIENTS

- 1 tbsp. essential olive oil
- 1 tbsp. Chopped cilantro
- 1 c. coconut milk
- 15 oz canned black beans, drained
- 1 lb. skinless and boneless chicken breasts
- 2 c. water
- ½ c. pumpkin flesh

NUTRITIONAL FACTS:

Calories: 254, Fat: 6 g, Carbs: 16 g, Protein: 22 g, Sodium: 92 mg

COOKING: 25'

PREPARATION: 15'

SERVES: 4

DIRECTIONS

1. Heat a pan when using oil over medium-high heat, add the chicken and cook for 5 minutes. Add the river, milk, pumpkin, and black beans toss, cover the pan, reduce heat to medium and cook for 20 mins. Add cilantro, toss, divide between plates and serve. Enjoy!

78. SPICY LAMB CURRY

INGREDIENTS

For Spice Mixture:

- 4 teaspoons ground coriander
- 4 teaspoons ground coriander
- 4 teaspoons ground cumin
- ¾ teaspoon ground ginger
- 2 teaspoons ground cinnamon
- ½ teaspoon ground cloves
- ½ teaspoon ground cardamom
- 2 tablespoons sweet paprika
- ½ tablespoon cayenne pepper
- 2 teaspoons chili powder
- 2 teaspoons salt

For Curry:

- 1 tablespoon coconut oil
- 2 pounds boneless lamb, trimmed and cubed into 1-inch size
- Salt and freshly ground black pepper, to taste
- 2 cups onions, chopped
- 1¼ cups water
- 1 cup coconut milk

NUTRITIONAL FACTS:

Calories: 183, Protein: 20 g, Fat: 4 g, Carbs: 24.5 g, Sodium: 87 mg

COOKING: 2H 45'

PREPARATION: 15'

SERVES: 6-8

DIRECTIONS

1. For spice mixture in a bowl, mix together all spices. Keep aside.
2. Season the lamb with salt and black pepper.
3. In a large Dutch oven, heat oil on medium-high heat.
4. Add lamb and stir fry for around 5 minutes.
5. Add onion and cook approximately 4-5 minutes.
6. Stir in spice mixture and cook approximately 1 minute.
7. Add water and coconut milk and provide to some boil on high heat.
8. Reduce the heat to low and simmer, covered for approximately 1-120 minutes or till desired doneness of lamb.
9. Uncover and simmer for approximately 3-4 minutes.
10. Serve hot.

79. GROUND LAMB WITH HARISSA

INGREDIENTS

- 1 tbsp. essential olive oil
- 1 tablespoon extra-virgin olive oil
- 2 red peppers, seeded and chopped finely
- 1 yellow onion, chopped finely
- 2 garlic cloves, chopped finely
- 1 teaspoon ground cumin
- ½ teaspoon ground turmeric
- ¼ teaspoon ground cinnamon
- ¼ teaspoon ground ginger
- 1½ pound lean ground lamb
- Salt, to taste
- 1 (14½-ounce) can diced tomatoes
- 2 tablespoons harissa
- 1 cup water
- Chopped fresh cilantro, for garnishing

NUTRITIONAL FACTS:

Calories: 168, Protein: 22 g, Fat: 8 g, Carbs: 16 g, Sodium: 147 mg

COOKING: 1H 11'

PREPARATION: 15'

SERVES: 4

DIRECTIONS

1. In a sizable pan, heat oil on medium-high heat.
2. Add bell pepper, onion and garlic and sauté for around 5 minutes.
3. Add spices and sauté for around 1 minute.
4. Add lamb and salt and cook approximately 5 minutes, getting into pieces.
5. Stir in tomatoes, harissa and water and provide with a boil.
6. Reduce the warmth to low and simmer, covered for about 1 hour.
7. Serve hot while using garnishing of harissa.

80. PAN-SEARED LAMB CHOPS

INGREDIENTS

- 4 garlic cloves, peeled
- Salt, to taste
- 1 teaspoon black mustard seeds, crushed finely
- 2 teaspoons ground cumin
- 1 teaspoon ground ginger
- 1 teaspoon ground coriander
- ½ teaspoon ground cinnamon
- Freshly ground black pepper, to taste
- 1 tablespoon coconut oil
- 8 medium lamb chops, trimmed

NUTRITIONAL FACTS:

Calories: 215, Protein: 24 g, Fat: 7 g, Carbs: 26 g, Sodium: 156 mg

COOKING: 4'-6'

PREPARATION: 10'

SERVES: 4

DIRECTIONS

1. Place garlic cloves onto a cutting board and sprinkle with a few salt.
2. With a knife, crush the garlic till a paste forms.
3. In a bowl, mix together garlic paste and spices.
4. With a clear, crisp knife, make 3-4 cuts on both side in the chops.
5. Rub the chops with garlic mixture generously.
6. In a large skillet, melt butter on medium heat.
7. Add chops and cook for approximately 2-3 minutes per side or till desired doneness.

81. LAMB & PINEAPPLE KEBABS

INGREDIENTS

- 1 large pineapple, cubed into 1½-inch size, divided
- 1 (½-inch) piece fresh ginger, chopped
- 2 garlic cloves, chopped
- Salt, to taste
- 16-24-ounce lamb shoulder steak, trimmed and cubed into 1½-inch size
- Fresh mint leaves coming from a bunch
- Ground cinnamon, to taste

NUTRITIONAL FACTS:

Calories: 159, Protein: 19 g, Fat: 6 g, Carbs: 11 g, Sodium: 99 mg

COOKING: 10'

PREPARATION: 15'

SERVES: 4-6

DIRECTIONS

1. In a blender, add about 1½ servings of pineapple, ginger, garlic and salt and pulse till smooth.
2. Transfer the amalgamation right into a large bowl.
3. Add chops and coat with mixture generously.
4. Refrigerate to marinate for about 1-2 hours.
5. Preheat the grill to medium heat. Grease the grill grate.
6. Thread lam, remaining pineapple and mint leaves onto pre-soaked wooden skewers.
7. Grill the kebabs approximately 10 min, turning occasionally.

82. SPICED PORK ONE

INGREDIENTS

- 1 (2-inch) piece fresh ginger, chopped
- 5-10 garlic cloves, chopped
- 1 teaspoon ground cumin
- ½ teaspoon ground turmeric 1 tablespoon hot paprika
- 1 tablespoon red pepper flakes
- Salt, to taste
- 2 tablespoons cider vinegar
- 2 pounds pork shoulder, trimmed and cubed into 1½-inch size
- 2 cups domestic hot water, divided
- 1 (1-inch wide) ball tamarind pulp
- ¼ cup olive oil
- 1 teaspoon black mustard seeds, crushed
- 4 green cardamoms
- 5 whole cloves
- 1 (3-inch) cinnamon stick
- 1 cup onion, chopped finely
- 1 large red bell pepper, seeded and chopped

NUTRITIONAL FACTS:

Calories: 138, Protein: 16 g, Fat: 8 g, Carbs: 17 g, Sodium: 118 mg

COOKING: 60'

PREPARATION: 15'

SERVES: 4

DIRECTIONS

1. In a food processor, add ginger, garlic, cumin, turmeric, paprika, red pepper flakes, salt and cider vinegar and pulse till smooth.
2. Transfer the amalgamation in to a large bowl.
3. Add pork and coat with mixture generously.
4. Keep aside, covered for around an hour at room temperature.
5. In a bowl, add 1 cup of warm water and tamarind and make aside till water becomes cool.
6. With the hands, crush the tamarind to extract the pulp.
7. Add remaining cup of hot water and mix till well combined.
8. Through a fine sieve, strain the tamarind juice inside a bowl.
9. In a sizable skillet, heat oil on medium-high heat.
10. Add mustard seeds, green cardamoms, cloves and cinnamon stick and sauté for about 4 minutes.
11. Add onion and sauté for approximately 5 minutes.
12. Add pork and stir fry for approximately 6 minutes.
13. Stir in tamarind juice and convey with a boil.
14. Reduce the heat to medium-low and simmer 1½ hours.
15. Stir in bell pepper and cook for about 7 minutes.

83. VEGETABLE CHEESE CALZONE

INGREDIENTS

- 3 asparagus stalks, cut into pieces
- 1/2 cup spinach, chopped
- 1/2 cup broccoli, chopped
- 1/2 cup sliced
- 2 tablespoons garlic, minced
- 2 teaspoons olive oil, divided
- 1/2 lb. frozen whole-wheat bread dough, thawed
- 1 medium tomato, sliced
- 1/2 cup mozzarella, shredded
- 2/3 cup pizza sauce

NUTRITIONAL FACTS:

Calories: 198, Fat: 8 g, Sodium: 124 mg, Carbs: 36 g, Protein: 12 g

COOKING: 20'

PREPARATION: 15'

SERVES: 4

DIRECTIONS

1. Prepare the oven to 400 degrees F to preheat. Grease a baking sheet with cooking oil and set it aside. Toss asparagus with mushrooms, garlic, broccoli, and spinach in a bowl. Stir in 1 teaspoon olive oil and mix well. Heat a greased skillet on medium heat.

2. Stir in vegetable mixture and sauté for 5 minutes. Set these vegetables aside. Cut the bread dough into quarters.

3. Spread each bread quarter on a floured surface into an oval. Add sautéed vegetables, 2 tbsp cheese, and tomato slice to half of each oval.

4. Wet the edges of each oval and fold the dough over the vegetable filling. Pinch and press the two edges.

5. Place these calzones on the baking sheet. Brush each calzone with foil and bake for 10 minutes. Heat pizza sauce in a saucepan for a minute. Serve the calzone with pizza sauce.

84. MIXED VEGETARIAN CHILI

INGREDIENTS

- 1 tablespoon olive oil
- 14 oz. canned black beans, rinsed and drained
- ½ cup yellow Onion, chopped
- 12 oz. extra-firm tofu, cut into pieces
- 14 oz. canned kidney beans, rinsed and drained
- 2 cans (14 oz.) diced tomatoes
- 3 tablespoons chili powder
- 1 tablespoon oregano
- 1 tablespoon chopped cilantro (fresh coriander)

NUTRITIONAL FACTS:

Calories: 314, Fat: 6 g, Sodium: 119 mg, Carbs: 46 g, Protein: 19 g

COOKING: 36'

PREPARATION: 10'

SERVES: 4

DIRECTIONS

1. Take a soup pot and heat olive oil in it over medium heat. Add onions and sauté for 6 minutes until soft. Add tomatoes, beans, chili powder, oregano, and beans. Boil it first, then reduce the heat to a simmer. Cook for 30 minutes, then add cilantro. Serve warm.

85. COCONUT CURRY SEA BASS

INGREDIENTS

- 1 can coconut milk
- Juice of 1 lime, freshly squeezed
- 1 tablespoon red curry paste
- 1 teaspoon coconut aminos
- 1 teaspoon honey
- 2 teaspoons sriracha
- 2 cloves of garlic, minced
- 1 teaspoon ground turmeric
- 1 tablespoon curry powder
- ¼ cup fresh cilantro
- Pepper

NUTRITIONAL FACTS:

Calories: 241.8, Carbs: 12.8 g, Protein: 3.1 g, Fats: 19.8 g, Sodium: 19 mg

COOKING: 15'

PREPARATION: 15'

SERVES: 3

DIRECTIONS

1. Place a heavy-bottomed pot on medium-high fire. Mix in all ingredients, then simmer on lower fire to a simmer and simmer for 5 minutes. Serve and enjoy.

86. ZUCCHINI PEPPER KEBABS

INGREDIENTS

- 1 small zucchini, sliced into 8 pieces
- 1 red onion, cut into 4 wedges
- 1 green bell pepper, cut into 4 chunks
- 8 cherry tomatoes
- 8 button mushrooms
- 1 red bell pepper, cut into 4 chunks
- 1/2 cup Italian dressing, fat-free
- 1/2 cup brown rice
- 1 cup of water
- 4 wooden skewers, soaked and drained

NUTRITIONAL FACTS:

Calories: 335, Fat: 8.2 g, Sodium: 516 mg, Carbs: 67 g, Protein: 8.8 g

COOKING: 40'

PREPARATION: 15'

SERVES: 2

DIRECTIONS

1. Toss tomatoes with zucchini, onion, peppers, and mushrooms in a bowl. Stir in Italian dressing and mix well to coat the vegetables. Marinate them for 10 minutes. Boil water with rice in a saucepan, then reduce the heat to a simmer.

2. Cover the rice and cook for 30 minutes until rice is done. Meanwhile, prepare the grill and preheat it on medium heat. Grease the grilling rack with cooking spray and place it 4 inches above the heat.

3. Thread 2 mushrooms, 2 tomatoes, and 2 zucchini slices along with 1 onions wedge, 1 green and red pepper slice on each skewer. Grill these kebabs for 5 minutes per side. Serve warm with boiled rice.

87. ASPARAGUS CHEESE VERMICELLI

INGREDIENTS

- 2 teaspoons olive oil, divided
- 6 asparagus spears, cut into pieces
- 4 oz. dried whole-grain vermicelli
- 1 medium tomato, chopped
- 1 tablespoon garlic, minced
- 2 tablespoons fresh basil, chopped
- 4 tablespoons Parmesan, freshly grated, divided
- 1/8 teaspoon black pepper, ground

NUTRITIONAL FACTS:

Calories: 325, Fat: 8 g, Sodium: 350 mg, Carbs: 48 g, Protein: 7.3 g

COOKING: 15'

PREPARATION: 10'

SERVES: 4

DIRECTIONS

1. Add 1 tsp oil to a skillet and heat it. Stir in asparagus and sauté until golden brown.

2. Cut the sautéed asparagus into 1-inch pieces. Fill a sauce pot with water up to ¾ full. After boiling the water, add pasta and cook for 10 minutes until it is all done.

3. Drain and rinse the pasta under tap water. Add pasta to a large bowl, then toss in olive oil, tomato, garlic, asparagus, basil, garlic, and parmesan. Serve with black pepper on top.

88. PESTO CHICKEN BREASTS WITH SUMMER SQUASH

INGREDIENTS

- 4 medium boneless, skinless chicken breast halves
- 1 tbsp. olive oil
- 2 tbsps. Homemade pesto
- 2 c. finely chopped zucchini
- 2 tbsps. Finely shredded Asiago

NUTRITIONAL FACTS:

Calories: 230, Fat: 9 g, Carbs: 8 g, Protein: 30 g, Sodium: 578 mg

COOKING: 10'

PREPARATION: 15'

SERVES: 4

DIRECTIONS

1. Cook your chicken in hot oil on medium heat within 4 minutes in a large nonstick skillet. Flip the chicken then put the zucchini.

2. Cook within 4 to 6 minutes more or until the chicken is tender and no longer pink (170 F), and squash is crisp-tender, stirring squash gently once or twice. Transfer chicken and squash to 4 dinner plates. Spread pesto over chicken; sprinkle with Asiago.

89. CHICKEN, TOMATO AND GREEN BEANS

INGREDIENTS

- 6 oz. low-sodium canned tomato paste
- 2 tbsps. Olive oil
- ¼ tsp. black pepper
- 2 lbs. trimmed green beans
- 2 tbsps. Chopped parsley
- 1 ½ lbs. boneless, skinless, and cubed chicken breasts
- 25 oz. no-salt-added canned tomato sauce

NUTRITIONAL FACTS:

Calories: 190, Fat: 4 g, Carbs: 12 g, Protein: 9 g, Sodium: 168 mg

COOKING: 25'

PREPARATION: 15'

SERVES: 4

DIRECTIONS

1. Heat a pan with 50 % with the oil over medium heat, add chicken, stir, cover, cook within 5 minutes on both sides and transfer to a bowl. Heat inside the same pan while using rest through the oil over medium heat, add green beans, stir and cook for 10 minutes.

2. Return chicken for that pan, add black pepper, tomato sauce, tomato paste, and parsley, stir, cover, cook for 10 minutes more, divide between plates and serve. Enjoy!

90. CHICKEN TORTILLAS

INGREDIENTS

- 6 oz. boneless, skinless, and cooked chicken breasts
- Black pepper
- 1/3 c. fat-free yogurt
- 4 heated up whole-wheat tortillas
- 2 chopped tomatoes

NUTRITIONAL FACTS:

Calories: 190, Fat: 2 g, Carbs: 12 g, Protein: 6 g, Sodium: 300 mg

COOKING: 5'

PREPARATION: 15'

SERVES: 4

DIRECTIONS

1. Heat-up a pan over medium heat, add one tortilla during those times, heat up, and hang them on the working surface. Spread yogurt on each tortilla, add chicken and tomatoes, roll, divide between plates and serve. Enjoy!

91. ROAST AND MUSHROOMS

INGREDIENTS

- 1 tsp. Italian seasoning
- 12 oz. low-sodium beef stock
- 3 1/2 lbs. pork roast
- 4 oz. sliced mushrooms

NUTRITIONAL FACTS:

Calories: 310, Fat: 16 g, Carbs: 10 g, Protein: 22 g, Sugars: 4 g, Sodium: 600 mg

COOKING: 20'

PREPARATION: 10'

SERVES: 4

DIRECTIONS

1. In a roasting pan, combine the roast with mushrooms, stock and Italian seasoning, and toss
2. Introduce inside the oven and bake at 350F for starters hour and 20 minutes.
3. Slice the roast, divide it along while using mushroom mix between plates and serve.
4. Enjoy!

92. PORK AND CELERY MIX

INGREDIENTS

- 3 tsps. Fenugreek powder
- Black pepper
- 1 tbsp. organic olive oil
- 1 1/2 c. coconut cream
- 26 oz. chopped celery leaves and stalks
- 1 lb. cubed pork meat
- 1 tbsp. chopped onion

NUTRITIONAL FACTS:

Calories: 340, Fat: 5 g, Carbs: 8 g, Protein: 14 g, Sugars: 2.1 g, Sodium: 200 mg

COOKING: 30'

PREPARATION: 10'

SERVES: 8

DIRECTIONS

1. Heat up a pan while using oil over medium-high heat, add the pork as well as the onion, black pepper and fenugreek, toss and brown for 5 minutes.

2. Add the celery too because coconut cream, toss, cook over medium heat for twenty minutes, divide everything into bowls and serve.

3. Enjoy!

93. CORN STUFFED PEPPERS

INGREDIENTS

- 4 red or green bell peppers
- 1 tablespoon olive oil
- ¼ cup onion, chopped
- 1 green bell pepper, chopped
- 2 1/2 cups fresh corn kernels
- 1/8 teaspoon chili powder
- 2 tablespoons chopped fresh parsley
- 3 egg whites
- 1/2 cup skim milk
- 1/2 cup water

NUTRITIONAL FACTS:

Calories: 197, Fat: 5 g, Sodium: 749 mg, Carbs: 29 g, Protein: 9 g

COOKING: 35'

PREPARATION: 10'

SERVES: 4

DIRECTIONS

1. Prepare the oven to 350 F to preheat. Layer a baking dish with cooking spray. Cut the bell peppers from the top and remove their seeds from inside. Put the peppers in your prepared baking dish with their cut side up.

2. Add oil to a skillet, then heat it on medium flame. Stir in onion, corn, and green pepper. Sauté for 5 minutes. Add cilantro and chili powder. Switch the heat to low. Mix milk plus egg whites in a bowl. Pour this mixture into the skillet and cook for 5 minutes while stirring.

3. Divide this mixture into each pepper. Add some water to the baking dish. Cover the stuffed peppers with an aluminum sheet. Bake for 15 minutes, then serves warm.

94. BLACK BEAN SOUP

INGREDIENTS

- 1-pound dried black beans, soaked overnight and rinsed
- 1 onion, chopped
- 1 carrot, peeled and chopped
- 2 jalapeño peppers, seeded and diced
- 6 cups Vegetable Broth or store-bought
- 1 teaspoon ground cumin
- 1 teaspoon ground coriander
- 1 teaspoon chili powder
- ½ teaspoon ground chipotle pepper
- ½ teaspoon of sea salt
- ¼ teaspoon freshly ground black pepper
- Pinch cayenne pepper
- ¼ cup fat-free sour cream, for garnish (optional)
- ¼ cup grated low-fat Cheddar cheese, for garnish (optional)

NUTRITIONAL FACTS:

Calories: 320, Fat: 3 g, Carbs: 57 g, Fiber: 13 g, Protein: 18 g, Sodium: 430 mg

COOKING: 8H

PREPARATION: 15'

SERVES: 6

DIRECTIONS

1. In your slow cooker, combine all the fixing listed, then cook on low for 8 hours. If you'd like, mash the beans with a potato masher, or purée using an immersion blender, blender, or food processor. Serve topped with the optional garnishes, if desired.

95. CHICKPEA & KALE SOUP

INGREDIENTS

- 1 summer squash, quartered lengthwise and sliced crosswise
- 1 zucchini, quartered lengthwise and sliced crosswise
- 2 cups cooked chickpeas, rinsed
- 1 cup uncooked quinoa
- 2 cans diced tomatoes, with their juice
- 5 cups Vegetable Broth, Poultry Broth, or store-bought
- 1 teaspoon garlic powder
- 1 teaspoon onion powder
- 1 teaspoon dried thyme
- ½ teaspoon of sea salt
- 2 cups chopped kale leaves

NUTRITIONAL FACTS:

Calories: 221, Fat: 3 g, Carbs: 40 g, Fiber: 7 g, Protein: 10 g, Sodium: 124 mg

COOKING: 9H

PREPARATION: 15'

SERVES: 6

DIRECTIONS

1. In your slow cooker, combine the summer squash, zucchini, chickpeas, quinoa, tomatoes (with their juice), broth, garlic powder, onion powder, thyme, and salt. Cover and cook on low within 8 hours. Stir in the kale. Cover and cook on low for 1 more hour.

96. CLAM CHOWDER

INGREDIENTS

- 1 red onion, chopped
- 3 carrots, peeled and chopped
- 1 fennel bulb and fronds, chopped
- 1 (10-ounce) can chopped clams, with their juice
- 1-pound baby red potatoes, quartered
- 4 cups Poultry Broth or store-bought
- ½ teaspoon of sea salt
- 1/8 teaspoon freshly ground black pepper
- 2 cups skim milk
- ¼ pound turkey bacon, browned and crumbled, for garnish

NUTRITIONAL FACTS:

Calories: 172, Fat: 1 g, Carbs: 29 g, Fiber: 4 g, Protein: 10 g, Sodium: 517 mg

COOKING: 8H

PREPARATION: 15'

SERVES: 6

DIRECTIONS

1. In your slow cooker, combine the onion, carrots, fennel bulb and fronds, clams (with their juice), potatoes, broth, salt, and pepper. Cover and cook on low within 8 hours. Stir in the milk and serve garnished with the crumbled bacon.

97. HONEY SPICED CAJUN CHICKEN

INGREDIENTS

- 2 chicken breasts, skinless, boneless
- 1 Tablespoon butter or margarine
- 1 pound of linguini
- 3 large mushrooms, sliced
- 1 large tomato, diced
- 2 Tablespoons regular mustard
- 4 Tablespoons honey
- 3 ounces low-fat table cream
- Parsley, roughly chopped

NUTRITIONAL FACTS:

Calories: 112, Protein: 12 g, Carbs: 56 g, Fat: 20 g, Sodium: 158 mg

COOKING: 20'

PREPARATION: 15'

SERVES: 4

DIRECTIONS

1. Wash and dry the chicken breasts. Warm 1 tablespoon of butter or margarine in a large pan. Add the chicken breasts. Season with salt and pepper. Cook on each side 6 – 10 minutes, until cooked thoroughly. Pull the chicken breasts from the pan. Set aside.

2. Cook the linguine as stated to instructions on the package in a large pot. Save 1 cup of the pasta water. Drain the linguine. Add the mushrooms, tomatoes to the pan from cooking the chicken. Heat until they are tender.

3. Add the honey, mustard, and cream. Combine thoroughly. Add the chicken and linguine to the pan. Stir until coated. Garnish with parsley. Serve immediately.

98. ITALIAN CHICKEN

INGREDIENTS

- 4 chicken breasts, skinless boneless
- 1 large jar of pasta sauce, low sodium
- 1 Tablespoon flavorless oil (olive, canola, or sunflower)
- 1 large onion, diced
- 1 large green pepper, diced
- ½ teaspoon garlic salt
- Salt and pepper to taste
- 1 cup low-fat mozzarella cheese, grated
- Spinach leaves, washed, dried, rough chop

NUTRITIONAL FACTS:

Calories: 142, Protein: 17 g, Carbs: 51 g, Fat: 15 g, Sodium: 225 mg

COOKING: 35'

PREPARATION: 15'

SERVES: 4

DIRECTIONS

1. Wash the chicken breasts, pat dry. In a large pot, heat the oil. Add the onion, cook, until it sweats and becomes translucent. Add the chicken. Season with salt, pepper, and garlic salt. Cook the chicken. 6 – 10 minutes on each side.

2. Add the peppers. Cook for 2 minutes. Pour the pasta sauce over the chicken. Mix well. Simmer on low for 20 minutes. Serve on plates, sprinkle the cheese over each piece. Garnish with spinach.

99. LEMON-PARSLEY CHICKEN BREAST

INGREDIENTS

- 2 chicken breasts, skinless, boneless
- 1/3 cup white wine
- 1/3 cup lemon juice
- 2 garlic cloves, minced
- 3 Tablespoons bread crumbs
- 2 Tablespoons flavorless oil (olive, canola, or sunflower)
- ¼ cup fresh parsley

NUTRITIONAL FACTS:

Calories: 117, Protein: 14 g, Carbs: 74 g, Fat: 12 g, Sodium: 189 mg

COOKING: 15'

PREPARATION: 15'

SERVES: 2

DIRECTIONS

1. Mix the wine, lemon juice, plus garlic in a measuring cup. Pound each chicken breast until they are ¼ inch thick. Coat the chicken with bread crumbs, and heat the oil in a large skillet.

2. Fry the chicken within 6 minutes on each side, until they turn brown. Stir in the wine mixture over the chicken. Simmer for 5 minutes. Pour any extra juices over the chicken. Garnish with parsley.

100. CURRANT PORK CHOPS

INGREDIENTS

- 2 Tablespoons Dijon Mustard
- 6 Pork Loin Chops, Center Cut
- 2 Teaspoons Olive Oil
- 1/3 Cup Wine Vinegar
- ¼ Cup Black Currant Jam
- 6 Orange Slices
- 1/8 Teaspoon Black Pepper

NUTRITIONAL FACTS:

Calories: 265, Protein: 25 g, Fat: 6 g, Carbs: 11 g, Sodium: 120 mg, Cholesterol: 22 mg

COOKING: 20'

PREPARATION: 10'

SERVES: 6

DIRECTIONS

1. Start by mixing your mustard and jam together in a bowl.

2. Get out a nonstick skillet, and grease it with olive oil before placing it over medium heat. Cook your chops for five minutes per side, and then top with a tablespoon of the jam mixture. Cover, and allow it to cook for two minutes. Transfer them to a serving plate.

3. Pour your wine vinegar in the same skillet, and scape the bits up to deglaze the pan, mixing well. Drizzle this over your pork chops.

4. Garnish with pepper and orange slices before serving warm.

CONCLUSION

Thank you for making it to the end. Initially, when the DASH diet was created, it was solely developed to reduce and stop the spread of hypertension, but it was later discovered that people who adopted the DASH diet were able to lose their weight to a considerable and moderate level. The reason for this was because of what the DASH diet entails that has made it effective for weight loss. As we end this book, here are some tips on how you can make your DASH diet work.

Remove processed and junk food from your refrigerator: With the DASH diet, eliminate that food from the refrigerator because they contain a high level of calories and unhealthy fats. Replace processed and junk foods with fresh fruits, vegetables, grains, and raw nuts. Throwing away the junk may seem too much to do; however, the best thing to do is refrain from buying them.

Prepare a grocery list: Before heading to the supermarket, ensure you have a list of the DASH diet food to purchase. This is to help to refrain from what is not on the grocery list in respect to the DASH diet

Prepare your meal whenever possible: No matter how sweet and healthy a meal prepared in the restaurant is, you don't know the combination of the ingredients, whether it is a detriment to your weight loss or not. It is therefore important to ensure you prepare your meal all by yourself most times, and by so doing, you can monitor what goes into your body regarding the DASH diet

Stock your kitchen with DASH food: To avoid the

temptation of eating foods that are detrimental to your weight loss, stock your kitchen with DASH food from time to time. By so doing, you get accustomed to the DASH diet

Avoid eating unhealthy snacks: Do away with snacks with unhealthy seasonings rather than go for snacks like popcorn cooked in olive oil and seasoned with garlic.

Consume less sodium: Food like bread, baked food, breakfast cereals, condiments, sauce, and canned products contain a high level of sodium, and these must be taken at the required level to avoid posing a danger to the bodyweight.

Checking of labels: Most people are victims of the act of not checking labels on food items purchased; thus, endangering their health. Check the labels of every food item in your kitchen and refrigerator and dispose of anything that has a high intake of sodium, sugar, white flour, saturated or trans fats.

Portion control and serving sizes: This involves eating a variety of food in the right proportion and getting the required amount of nutrients needed. Eating to get overfed is what most people do, all for the sake of eating to one's satisfaction; with this simple act, most people don't know that obesity can be gotten this, thus with the DASH diet, individuals know the amount of food to be taken with regards to the normal body functioning system and thereby having a balanced body weight.

Avoid Sedentary habit: This is a lifestyle that involves little or no physical activities. Examples of sedentary lifestyles are sitting with the computer all day long, reading all day long, or watching television most hours of the day. This kind of habit is not encouraged in the DASH diet, thereby not leading to unnecessary weight gain—more of a reason why the DASH diet encourages physical exercise.

I hope you have learned something!

INDEX

A

Almond Butter-Banana Smoothie; 49

Apple & Berry Cobbler; 238

Apple Pancakes; 75

Apple Quinoa Muffins; 127

Apricot Biscotti; 237

Artichoke and Spinach Chicken; 248

Asian Pork Tenderloin; 205

Asian Salmon; 141

Asparagus Cheese Vermicelli; 265

Avocado Cup with Egg; 37

B

Bagels Made Healthy; 180

Baked Chicken; 149

Baked Fish Served with Vegetables; 43

Banana & Cinnamon Oatmeal; 139

Banana Bread; 230

Banana-Peanut Butter and Greens Smoothie; 167

Basil Halibut; 91

Beef Stew with Fennel and Shallots; 68

Black Bean Soup; 272

Black Bean Stew with Cornbread; 62

Blueberry Oat Muffins; 229

Blueberry Waffles; 102

Blueberry-Vanilla Yogurt Smoothie; 166

Breakfast Banana Split; 111

Breakfast Fruits Bowls; 115; 176

Brown Sugar Cinnamon Oatmeal; 45

C

Carrot Cake Overnight Oats; 147

Carrot Muffins; 66

Cereal with Cranberry-Orange Twist; 181

Chia Seeds Breakfast Mix; 175

Chicken Thighs and Apples Mix; 200

Chicken Tortillas; 268

Chicken with Mushrooms; 55

Chicken with Potatoes Olives & Sprouts; 153

Chicken Wrap; 42

Chicken, Tomato and Green Beans; 267

Chickpea & Kale Soup; 274

Chickpea Cauliflower Tikka Masala; 84

Clam Chowder; 274

Cobb Pasta Salad; 210

Coconut Curry Sea Bass; 262

Coconut Shrimp; 125

Corn Stuffed Peppers; 271

Creamy Apple-Avocado Smoothie; 158

Creamy Avocado and Egg Salad Sandwiches; 184

Creamy Haddock with Kale; 219

Creamy Oats & Blueberry Smoothie; 93

Currant Pork Chops; 279

Curried Beef Meatballs; 198

Curry Vegetable Noodles with Chicken; 58

D

Dill and Lemon Cod Packets; 72

Dill Chicken Salad; 94

E

Easy Beef Brisket; 39

Easy Lunch Salmon Steaks; 120

Easy Pork Chops; 195

Easy Shrimp; 86

Easy Steamed Alaskan Cod; 128

Easy Veggie Muffins; 119

Edamame Salad with Corn and Cranberries; 211

Egg White Breakfast Mix; 152

Eggplant Parmesan Stacks; 67

Energy Sunrise Muffins; 88

F

Falling "Off" The Bone Chicken; 202

Fish Amandine; 192

Fish in A Vegetable Patch; 133

French Toast with Applesauce; 172

Fruited Quinoa Salad; 116

G

Garlic and Tomatoes on Mussels; 245

Garlic Mushroom Chicken; 38

Garlic Pepper Chicken; 145

Garlic Pork Shoulder; 203

Generous Garlic Bread Stick; 241

Ginger Sesame Salmon; 154

Greek Yogurt Oat Pancakes; 41

Grilled Flank Steak with Lime Vinaigrette; 204

Grilled Pork Fajitas; 117

Ground Beef with Greens & Tomatoes; 196

Ground Lamb with Harissa; 252

H

Honey Crusted Chicken; 77

Honey Spiced Cajun Chicken; 276

I

Italian Chicken; 277

Italian Stuffed Portobello Mushroom Burgers; 54

L

Lamb & Pineapple Kebabs; 256

Leek & Cauliflower Soup; 100

Lemon Garlic Shrimp; 190

Lemon Salmon with Kaffir Lime; 193

Lemongrass and Chicken Soup; 112

Lemon-Parsley Chicken Breast; 278

Light Balsamic Salad; 108

M

Mexican-Style Potato Casserole; 90

Milk Chocolate Pudding; 232

Mini Teriyaki Turkey Sandwiches; 222

Minty Lime and Grapefruit Yogurt Parfait; 233

Mixed Fruit Compote Cups; 240

Mixed Vegetarian Chili; 261

Mushrooms and Cheese Omelet; 123

Mustard Chicken Tenders; 109

N

No Cook Overnight Oats; 182

O

Oatmeal Banana Pancakes with Walnuts; 57

Olive Capers Chicken; 59

Oven-Fried Chicken Breasts; 246

P

Paella with Chicken, Leeks, and Tarragon; 47
Pan-Seared Lamb Chops; 254
Peach Crumble Muffins; 223
Peach Tarts; 234
Peanut Butter Banana Bread Bites; 225
Pesto Chicken Breasts with Summer Squash; 266
Pesto Omelet; 179
Pineapple Oatmeal; 135
Pork and Celery Mix; 270
Pork and Dates Sauce; 132
Pork and Roasted Tomatoes Mix; 81
Pork Medallions with Five Spice Powder; 104
Pork Roast and Cranberry Roast; 194
Provence Pork Medallions; 121
Pumpkin and Black Beans Chicken; 249
Pumpkin Cookies; 177
Pumpkin Muffins; 71

R

Raspberry Nuts Parfait; 236
Roast and Mushrooms; 269
Rosemary Roasted Chicken; 247
Rustic Beef and Barley Soup; 207

S

Salmon Wrap; 76
Salsa Chicken Chili; 51
Savory Lobster Roll; 244

Savory Yogurt Bowls; 53

Scrambled Egg and Veggie Breakfast Quesadillas; 83

Seared Scallops with Blood Orange Glaze; 189

Shrimp Fra Diavolo; 191

Simple Beef Brisket and Tomato Soup; 129; 206

Simple Cheese and Broccoli Omelets; 183

Southwestern Bean Salad with Creamy Avocado Dressing; 209

Southwestern Chicken and Pasta; 64

Southwestern Vegetables Tacos; 188

Spiced Pork One; 257

Spicy Cod; 113

Spicy Lamb Curry; 250

Spicy Tofu Burrito Bowls with Cilantro Avocado Sauce; 148

Spinach, Egg, And Cheese Breakfast Quesadillas; 97; 98

Steamed Blue Crabs; 137

Steamed Fish with Scallions and Ginger; 217

Steamed Salmon Teriyaki; 103

Steamed Tilapia with Green Chutney; 218

Steamed Veggie and Lemon Pepper Salmon; 216

Steel Cut Oat Blueberry Pancakes; 131

Steel-Cut Oatmeal with Plums and Pear; 171

Stewed Cod Filet with Tomatoes; 220

Strawberry Sandwich; 79

Strawberry, Orange, and Beet Smoothie; 159

Stuffed Chicken Breasts; 73

Stuffed Eggplant Shells; 186

Super-Simple Granola; 107

Sweet and Sour Chicken Whit Noodles and Vegetables; 98

Sweet Berries Pancake; 61

Sweet Potato Toast Three Ways; 170

Sweet Potatoes and Zucchini Soup; 80

Sweet Potato-Turkey Meatloaf; 136
Sweet-Ginger Scallops; 243

T

Tangy Three-Bean Salad with Barley; 213
Thai Chicken Thighs; 201
Toasted Almond Ambrosia; 227
Tofu & Green Bean Stir-Fry; 50
Tuna Salad-Stuffed Tomatoes with Arugula; 215
Tuna Sandwich; 46
Turkey Wrap; 140

V

Vegetable Cheese Calzone; 259
Veggie Scramble; 178
Very Berry Muesli; 169

W

Warm Asian Slaw; 212
White Beans Stew; 144
White Beans with Spinach and Pan-Roasted Tomatoes; 95
White Chicken Chili; 124

Z

Zesty Zucchini Muffins; 228
Zucchini Pancakes; 143
Zucchini Pepper Kebabs; 263

Manufactured by Amazon.ca
Bolton, ON